What a wonderful culmination of two decades ⌐▫▫▫▫▫ people with Alzheimer's dementia. *Alzheimer's 911* is an impressive, empowering, and honest book, full of frank and fearless advice and very practical help. Frena draws from her widely varied real-life experience as an Alzheimer's dementia caregiver and walks you through step-by-step. This is a must-read guidebook, covering all aspects of dementia care from Alzheimer's to the many other dementias of age. Her personal anecdotes are both touching and humorous, and she enables caregivers to understand what is really going on inside the person with dementia. I have to say I laughed and I cried and found this book very entertaining, as well as deeply spiritual. This is one Alzheimer's book you don't have to be afraid to pick up!

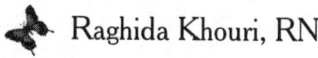 Raghida Khouri, RN

Frena Gray-Davidson's *Alzheimer's 911* is an indispensable gift to anyone dealing with dementia. With humor, sensitivity and clarity, the author flawlessly offers the two most profound and precious tools to anyone associated with dementia diseases: Hope and Pragmatism.

As most of us have sadly discovered, hope and Alzheimer's are rarely used together in the same sentence; but in her book, Frena makes the compelling and life-saving case that a rich, meaningful life can indeed be an integral part of the Alzheimer's process. And after making that assertion, she provides practical, concrete, step-by-step pointers for how to achieve precisely such a worthy life while on the Alzheimer's journey. . . whether as afflicted or caregiver.

Frena delivers convincingly and wholeheartedly on her promise to not only make your journey bearable, but to teach you that, in fact, the journey itself will bear you up. For any on the Alzheimer's path, I can only urge them to do themselves the ultimate favor: Read, follow and enjoy this book!

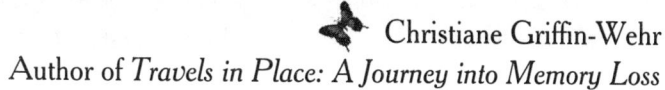 Christiane Griffin-Wehr
Author of Travels in Place: A Journey into Memory Loss

If you are a caregiver, if you are a friend to a caregiver, you need to read *Alzheimer's 911*. If you are a pastor, you need to keep many copies of this book within reach of your favorite translation of the Bible. When church members find the courage to tell you of their struggles with a family member or a spouse, you will have a poignant, fun, and realistic resource that will guide them and offer encouragement and simple insight into this caregiving adventure.

Frena Gray-Davidson gives us a fresh way to walk through this holy ground of caregiving. She opens a window that does not show a brick wall but a colorful garden of possibility. Frena has led a lively caregiver support group at our church for a number of years. No one leaves empty. When their well runs dry, they show up...again and again.

Alzheimer's 911 turns the horrendous word "victimhood" into "transformation." It offers creative, profound, and simple ways of being on this journey together, no longer as strangers but as friends.

I have known Frena for eight years. When I moved to Sierra Vista, AZ, my mother was in "Alzheimer's Land." I had read plenty of information on medical advances. I was tired of medical advances. What I needed as a daughter was to hear of the soul journey. I needed to hear a fresh perspective on caregiving that related to the heart and not the mind.

This book affirms the goal to be simple and profound as we encounter caregiving. It provides new ways of listening and laughing and thinking "outside the box." She offers candid illustrations of ways we can go about caregiving in fresh and creative ways. She names the ways we have been patronizing out of fear rather than out of compassion and peace.

Frena says it best: "Take the deeper, more profound, more deeply spiritual approach, and live your life in the present moment." Then our mothers, fathers, sisters, and brothers will know they are being listened to as you care for them. And you will know the transforming reality of "God with you" as you do the sacred work of caring for another.

Had I read *Alzheimer's 911* when my mother was in "Alzheimer's Land," I would have said, "Alleluia! This is hope. This is what caregiving is all about!"

Rev. Virginia Studer
Faith Presbyterian Church, Sierra Vista, AZ

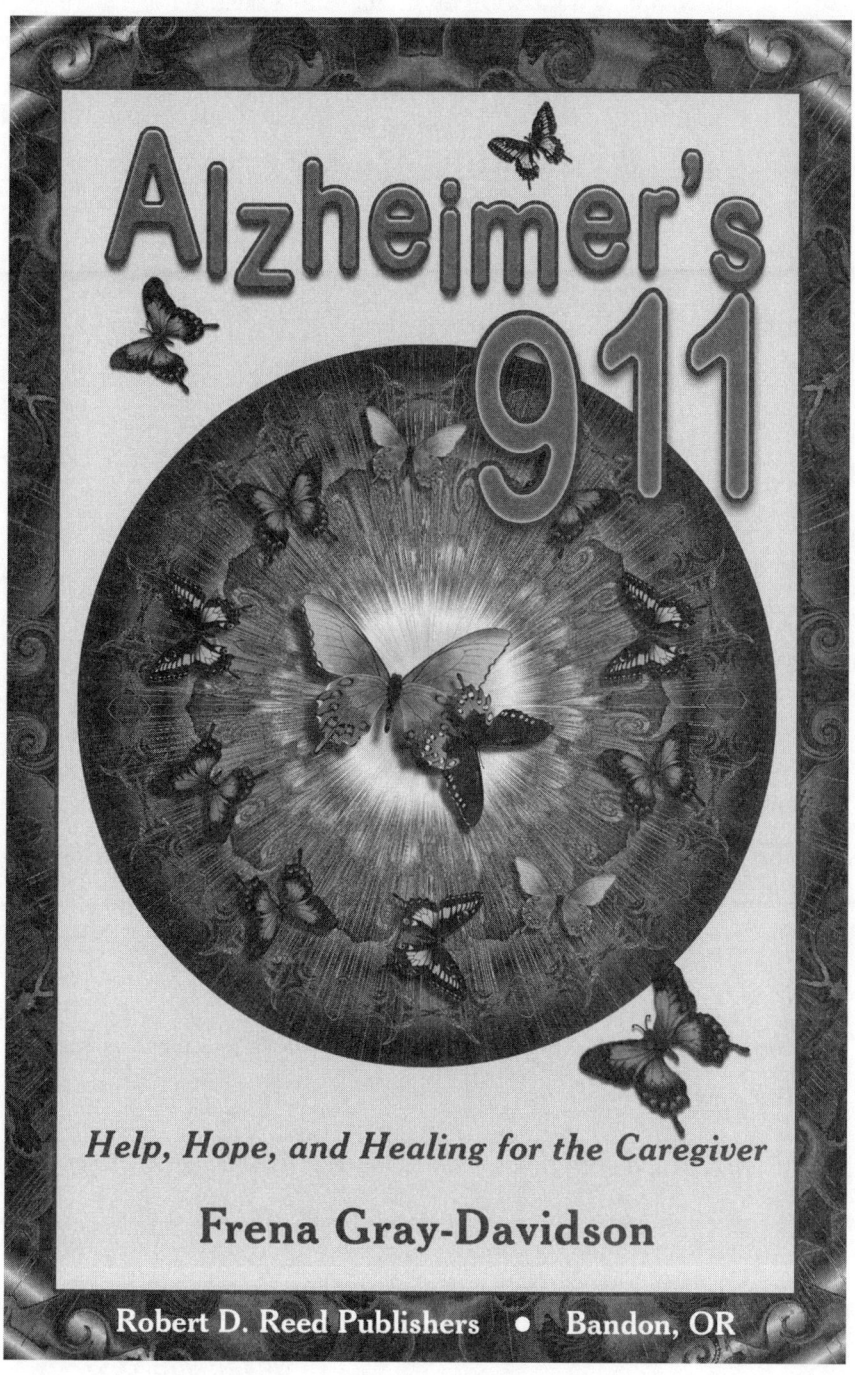

Alzheimer's 911

Help, Hope, and Healing for the Caregiver

Frena Gray-Davidson

Robert D. Reed Publishers • Bandon, OR

Robert D. Reed Publishers
P.O. Box 1992
Bandon, OR 97411
Phone: 541-347-9882; Fax: -9883
E-mail: 4bobreed@msn.com
Website: www.rdrpublishers.com

Editor: Kate Rakini
Cover Designer: Cleone L. Reed
Interior Book Designer: Amy Cole

ISBN: 978-1-934759-14-1

Library of Congress Control Number: 2009920089

Manufactured, Typeset, and Printed in the United States of America

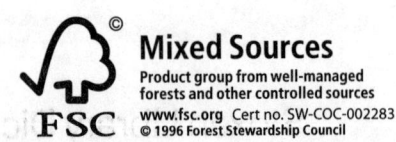

Mixed Sources

Product group from well-managed forests and other controlled sources
www.fsc.org Cert no. SW-COC-002283
© 1996 Forest Stewardship Council

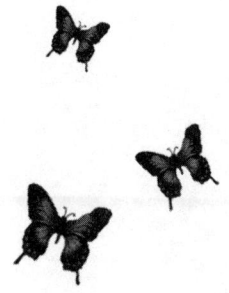

Dedication

This book is dedicated to my caregiving friends in Bisbee:

Myrtle Attaway, ninety-one and counting, who has cared for her parents, her husband, her friends, her many dogs – including her present faithful companion, Star – and blesses us with the best laugh in the world.

And to my dear friends Yvonne Grimm and Nancy Williams, caregivers to beloved husbands.

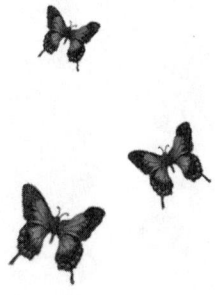

Acknowledgements

Alzheimer's caregiving is a fairly mentorless world, but, thank goodness, there has been Dr. Tom Kitwood, who truly taught that people with dementia are just as real and human as the rest of us and led the ground-breaking Bradford Dementia Project.

And there is the American Alzheimer's Association, the Alzheimer Society of Canada, and the Alzheimer Society of Great Britain – without whose support groups no caregiver would be sane.

In writing this book, I want to thank Dr. Georgia Neff, for invaluable information on the nutritional approach to the dementias, and Dr. Helen Saul, for research and information gathering.

I also want to thank Robert and Cleone Reed for their encouragement to write this book to meet the real inner-journey needs of caregivers.

Grateful thanks also to my wonderful editor, Kate Rakini, for patient help and good guidance.

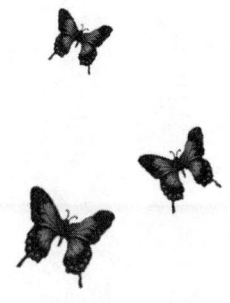

Table of Contents

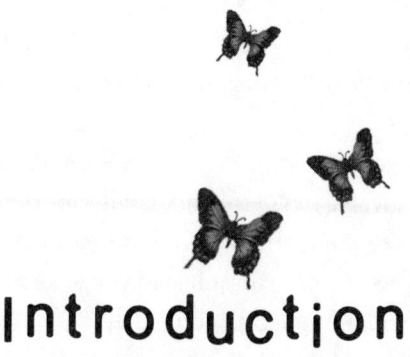

Introduction

Are You Feeling Crazy?

So you're dealing with Alzheimer's and it's making you crazy. Well, there's nothing wrong with you. Alzheimer's and most other dementias make most people feel that way at least three times a week. Welcome to the confusing world of dementia caregiving!

Now here's the good news. In spite of everything you've heard, you can make sense of all this. This book will teach you how. You don't have to stay confused, upset, angry, depressed, and feeling helpless. I can't promise you there will never be a day when you don't feel those things. However, if you build your understanding, practice your handling skills, nurture your own inner life, *and* make a really good self-care plan, you will be able to take charge of both caregiving and yourself.

Right now, we can't really fix Alzheimer's. However, it is currently the most researched disease on the planet, so you can rightly hope for a cure to be found literally at any moment. The good news is – you can fix you, and I'm here to help you do that.

Yet caregiving isn't about fixing anything. It's about creating a life you can bear and which, in turn, bears you. From the beginning, we are going to assume that you could make sense of everything in the world of dementia – if you only knew how. I'm going to teach you how. There are things you need to know about Alzheimer's that no one is telling you.

In fact, since the current fashion is to despair about Alzheimer's, any potentially good news tends to be withheld. For example, there is actually a meaningful inner journey going on inside the person who has dementia. There are important ways that a person with Alzheimer's may grow and develop in spite of their disease.

Daily happiness is very possible, even with Alzheimer's. And such happiness is also available for caregivers. It doesn't matter if you didn't want to become a caregiver. It doesn't even matter if you don't particularly like the person you are caregiving. This journey can still lead you to growth, forgiveness, and peace – if you are willing to accept some help.

That, my friend, is where I come in. Nothing you learn on this journey is wasted. Everything will enhance who you are, who you may become, and how you may grow. The whole secret of dealing with Alzheimer's is finding ways to answer the great spiritual question: "How am I being asked to grow?"

Being a caregiver is not a waste of time, even if you don't want to do it. Every task you learn, every dilemma you solve, every tear you wipe away – even if it's your own – and everything you forgive will expand your heart, your soul, and your whole being. It will bring to you a whole range of profound skills and gifts that can be applied to all the situations of your life.

It's okay if you don't believe me now. Just read this book one section at a time. Then try the techniques one at a time. Use the approaches suggested here and see what works and what doesn't in your particular situation.

I've been working with people with dementia for twenty years now. Maybe like you, I never intended to do such work. I was raised in England with parents who were both nurses by profession and, I can tell you, that was on top of the list of work I never intended to do. Caregiving never held any attraction for me. No, I wanted adventure.

So, I became a journalist and worked in Asia as a travel writer and broadcaster, traveling almost everywhere between India and China. Studied acupuncture and Chinese medicine. Practiced Buddhist meditation. Did Tai Chi in Hong Kong for five years with a great martial arts teacher. In short, had the kind of adventures I'd dreamed of.

Eventually I moved to America in search of what shaped the wonderful, lively, heart-centered Americans I'd met all over Asia. And yes, I wanted to grow myself more, too, though I wasn't clear how. But one thing I could have told you then, for absolute certain, was that being an Alzheimer's caregiver would not have been my choice. I never would have picked that as my pathway of development.

However, it picked me. As far as I was concerned, I was only looking to save some rent money when I moved into a shared house in Berkeley, California, to help care for a seventy-nine-year-old woman with a disease I couldn't spell and had never heard of. It was Alzheimer's, of course, and that was such a totally heart-changing time for me and my soul and spirit that I plunged into being an Alzheimer's caregiver for the next twenty years.

What's the difference between you and me? Am I, unlike you, a perfect caregiver unruffled in any way by the problems of caregiving? Oh please, let's get serious here! Ask anyone who knows me and they'll tell you the word "perfection" does not describe the average day of being me.

However, there probably is an important difference between you and me, and that is exactly what allowed me to learn what I have learned. The difference is that I had never heard of Alzheimer's before becoming a caregiver. That meant I had no preconceptions about it, leaving me free to be open and inventive. Nor have I been related to the people I've cared for. In my first experience, I had never met Hannah when she was healthy, so I wasn't upset by her losses. I also had three other helpers in the house, so I wasn't alone with the issues of caregiving.

When I began being an Alzheimer's caregiver, I went to several workshops and seminars. I found them largely useless. They seemed to be about brain cells, drugs, DNA – and despair. I knew I couldn't learn anything helpful in all of that. The nearest real help that I found was in the caregiver support groups offered by the Alzheimer's Association. For the first time I experienced real caregiving being talked about by real people actually doing the job, just like me. Unlike me, they were also dealing with sadness, loss, and the pain of watching someone they once knew become a completely different person.

I realized right then, in my first support group meeting, the essential difference between family caregivers and myself. It was like the difference between Fred Astaire and Ginger Rogers. You know the joke – she had to do everything he did, but wearing high heels and dancing backwards. In caregiving, I'm Fred Astaire and family caregivers are Ginger Rogers. That doesn't mean, however, that many of the things I learned can't be very useful to you. Because of my lower stress level and my lack of personal grief and pain, I was able to learn what I can now pass on to you.

It also helped that for the previous fifteen years in Asia I spent long periods of time in Nepal, Indonesia, India, and Hong Kong. Each one of those cultures was new to me when I arrived for the first time. I had to learn something of the language, the customs, and the lifestyle of each place in order to manage daily life at all.

Everywhere there were kind people willing and ready to help me get to know their world. I loved Asia and it was a very magical time in my life. Those experiences helped me understand that learning about Alzheimer's was going to be like learning about any other new culture. All my instincts told me that I should learn about Alzheimer's from the person I was caring for.

I knew I shouldn't listen to most so-called experts, especially if they only peddled hopelessness and despair. No, I knew intuitively that the Alzheimer's expert in our house was an elderly woman living in the midst of the disease – in Alzheimer Land, as I soon thought of it. There was no point in going to seminars that didn't empower me. Instead, I spent my time hanging out with a seventy-nine-year-old German Jewish refugee in Berkeley, California, and she became my Ph.D. in Alzheimer's.

The first year I didn't even realize how much I learned. My view of what was going on was so profoundly different from the mainstream medical view, and still is, that back then I doubted my own observations. It took me nine more years to understand what a wonderful teacher she had been, she and the others I cared for in those years. In that first decade, I had plenty of time to try out the many things I'm going to share with you. In the second decade of my Alzheimer's and dementia work, I began teaching families and professional caregivers what I had learned. It was, and is, all about developing relationships with people with dementia.

That, you see, is the heart of our struggle. How do we create a heartfelt relationship with someone made new to us because of an illness? An illness, moreover, that has changed this person into someone we don't want that person to be? No one wants someone close to them to change into a person with Alzheimer's or a similar dementia. Not only is the disease challenging enough as it is, but our society hates and fears it.

Caregivers are not being encouraged to learn the possibilities that still remain, which leaves us stuck with nothing but loss. If we liked this person before, how can we get over the change in them? If we didn't like this person much before, how on earth do we get over ourselves? Even worse, how do we make a heartfelt relationship with ourselves when we may not like ourselves as caregivers? If we are confused, grieving, angry, and distressed by demands, which promise to be endless, how can we find ways to like ourselves? These feel like insurmountable problems.

We can only change ourselves with tools, time, a willingness to grow, and the acceptance of a real but very different relationship in present time with this person who has dementia.

So in this book, we'll start with the easiest item – the tools. Then we'll get to some other useful things. Let me warn you – when it comes to dementia, there is nothing that always works. What works on a Tuesday afternoon may not work on a Friday morning, this week. Next week, who knows?

That's why you need a whole repertoire of approaches, skills, tricks, and devices in your box of tools. You need flexibility and ways to bribe, persuade, and manipulate. You need to grow a kind understanding of yourself and also of this person you caregive. Also – trust me on this – you really need to come to a place of secure love for yourself and others. Love is going to be your greatest management tool.

We do Alzheimer's caregiving just one day at a time and, some days, just one hour at a time. That's how we make it work. You'll succeed by developing new skills every day and trying them out repeatedly. Flexibility is your lifeline, and rigidity will break you in health and heart and will profoundly affect the one you care for.

So, let's find a way out of the craziness and into the light. First, we have to get on the Alzheimer's bus, where we'll start by throwing away almost every assumption our society makes about Alzheimer's, because they really aren't true.

For example, did you know that our modern Alzheimer's disease of today is not actually the disease studied by Dr. Alzheimer, nor is it much like the disease that was named after him by his director? He was not studying the dementia of old age, but something then called "pre-senile dementia."

We also assume that Alzheimer's disease affects people in ways it doesn't. We commonly describe people with Alzheimer's as empty and gone away, and it is widely assumed that nothing positive could possibly be going on within this disease. Even professional care people think this way.

They need, instead, to ask themselves whether their patients have gone away because there is nothing worth being present for. My experience of Alzheimer's is that people are present and reachable as we love and accept them for being exactly who they are. In that place, there are all kinds of activities they respond to and ways they can express themselves.

The heart and spirit of a person does not get Alzheimer's and may even recover from former wounding through the course of their disease. We assume their behaviors demonstrate dementia and that therefore they are meaningless disease symptoms. We don't see these behaviors as meaningful communications.

We create our own problems with dementia by choosing to see it as a battle of conflicting interests – our normal thinking versus the abnormal thinking of the person with dementia. That is how we start to make ourselves crazy and the person we care for lonely.

Listen to any medical description of Alzheimer's and all you hear is medical jargon about disease process. You don't hear much about people. Yet, it is only in looking inside the disease that we can find the person. It is only in finding that person within that we can find answers, for both of us. No one is a disease. A person is a person and may have a disease, which complicates living, but it does not dehumanize them. Be very suspicious of anyone who thinks that way, because they neither truly know people with dementia nor have answers for you. We would have known a great deal more about how to help, support, and reach people with dementia well before now if they had not been devalued.

Our main job is to learn how to be good caregivers. Until we care for ourselves as caregivers, we never successfully grow to the task. Instead, we'll become those angry, over-stressed, resentful people so often found in Alzheimer's caregiving. Much of this overall negativity comes from the inner being of the caregiver, not from the illness being dealt with.

On the whole, we have not asked dementia caregivers to learn the disease. We have not asked them to learn about themselves as caregivers and to take on the task of dealing with their own emotional and spiritual growth.

That is what this book asks of you. Learn the disease, discover yourself as a caregiver, and take the necessary steps to transform that within you that needs to be changed. Don't worry if you don't yet know how. That's why I wrote this book, so you can shorten your own distress period by learning from my mistakes. You'll also have many opportunities to learn from your own mistakes. And, I promise you, with your more flexible attitude, you'll have a lot more fun than all those people terrified of Alzheimer's.

Our society almost gloats about how overwhelmingly awful it is to be an Alzheimer's caregiver. I know many who have managed the task with grace, humor, and resilience – which doesn't mean they managed every single day with all of those qualities. Here's a starter list for growing yourself:

- Have the willingness to get to know the disease.
- Show openness to re-learning this person who now is affected by dementia.
- Practice the ability to sit in the present moment with this person.
- Develop the patience to take life slowly.
- Nurture compassion and love for someone on the dementia path.
- Cultivate forgiveness – of yourself, of others, and especially of the person you care for.

We caregivers can easily become addicted to problems, especially once we get tired, overwhelmed, upset, sleep-deprived, and emotionally drained. It's like any other addiction. We know where we are, what it feels like, and how familiar it is, so we put up with the pain of the addiction rather than take the challenge to grow and heal.

This book is about how caregivers can, and indeed must, grow spiritually and emotionally, in order to heal and free ourselves from pain in our caregiving lifestyle and to bring the best to the one we care for. It centers solely on the caregiving issues and the caregiver. It is a book about walking the caregiver walk in companionship with one who needs us. Once you learn that, you will have a much better time and so will the one you care for.

As we go forward, I want to share the story of how I first learned Alzheimer's from an expert living within the disease. An essay about this journey, "A Life in Alzheimer's Land," is interspersed throughout this book. I suggest that you, too, might find it helpful to journal about your own experiences of learning, struggling, and growing into the task of becoming a caregiver – especially the journey to relearn who this person has now become, hidden within dementia. So, let's go.

A LIFE IN ALZHEIMER'S LAND

I met Hannah and liked her immediately. She was sitting on a battered sofa and, when I sat down beside her, I held out my hand to her.

"Hallo, Hannah," I said. She took it between her own and held onto it. Her skin was soft and dry against mine and she looked at me out of light blue eyes, not old like the rest of her. She smiled. It started in her eyes, spread to her mouth, and slowly travelled until it filled her whole face with pleasure. I could feel the same big smile on my face. Then we both laughed. We had connected.

"It's so good that you came," she said, as if she had been waiting especially for me. Hannah welcomed me effortlessly into her heart. She was a dignified woman with a graciousness that survived her losses. Her understanding of the world around her was fractured and it gave her a bizarre charm.

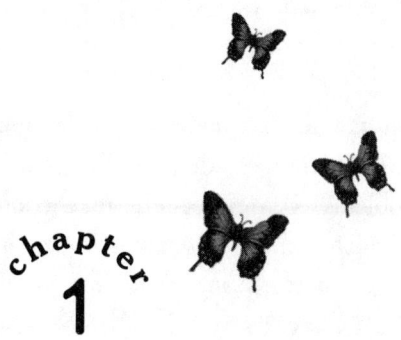

Starting Your Journey

I want to start by pointing out that I use the terms Alzheimer's and dementia interchangeably. Not only because Alzheimer's is actually one form of dementia, but also because, right or wrong, I have concluded that it is likely that we use the word Alzheimer's far too often. As I detail later, there is ample reason to note that causes have been found for the development of many dementias. Therefore, there is little reason to assume they are Alzheimer's dementia, when so far that remains a dementia of unknown cause, origin, and treatment.

Mine is not the usual view and I only come to it through observation of real people and their lives. I do not dissect brain cells or autopsy brains. I observe people with dementia, their lives, and the events of their lives and find they often have common pathways. I was the first observer ever to draw attention to the pattern of early serious deprivation in childhood among those later diagnosed with dementia.

At this point, I am the only person I know to suggest the use of digestive enzymes to improve brain function through more efficient absorption and distribution of nutrients — again based on personal observation. I may also be one of the few to suggest that the behaviors of dementia are meaningful communications rather than meaningless symptoms.

Agreeing with me doesn't matter. What matters is that you take your own learning in hand and trust your own observations while being with and caring for your person with dementia. You are your own expert and what you see is what you see. From what you see, you can make a care plan that works for both of you.

So I use Alzheimer's and dementia interchangeably for two reasons. One, because we lack the knowledge and genuine evidence to differentiate the dementias. Two, because our problems as caregivers are, for the most part, essentially the same, no matter which dementia we are dealing with. There may be subtle degrees of difference between the dementias, but the greater and more important differences for caregivers involve the usual range of idiosyncrasies between human beings. Everyone does dementia in his or her own way and that's what we have to learn. We have to learn each individual person and how their needs communicate themselves to us, if we are paying attention.

Family caregivers of elders with dementia often get stuck when they don't want to admit that life has changed and will never be the same again. Be willing to learn what the usual, normal, average symptoms of dementia are. See how they apply to your person. That way, you will save yourself tons of frustration, anger, resentment, and negativity. Even if you even slightly suspect that your mother or your mate is doing certain things to annoy you, a person who wanted to stay sane would be wise to attribute them all to dementia. Give it to the disease rather than the person.

One thing you can know for sure. If a person can get up in the morning with the sure intention of doing certain things to make you crazy, they don't have dementia. So if your man or your mom is driving you crazy, it's just by happy accident, not by successful intention. The other really important part of getting to know dementia is that people really can grow and develop even in the midst of their losses.

Getting to Know Dementia

I have observed that people with Alzheimer's have almost invariably had difficult childhoods and have often grown up to be fearful, wounded, anxious, secretive, or angry. They were wounded long ago and such wounds can hurt forever. People get very used to their own pain and discomfort and do not realize that the wound is not in their hearts. The wound is centered in their defense system, and that comes from the mind, *not* from the heart.

If you don't actually believe this right now, that's okay. It's a fairly radical idea and one that I learned entirely from people with dementia. I always thought my feelings, defenses, and wounds were, of course, centered in my heart. Being with people with dementia for so long, I noticed that as they lost their relationship with reliable memory and the meaning of their own feelings, they often became very different people.

At first, they found peace, and then they moved to joyfulness, a sense of play, and even into a sort of blissfulness. Our deepest heart-centered feelings are always joy and love. When mind can no longer control the gates of the heart with fear or anger, people can then enter the sacred space where absolute love and joy reside. Alzheimer's and the other dementias can open the heart in a whole new way as memory and early training loosen their hold. People can become happy, unworried, less fearful, and much more loving. It is not at all uncommon in the progress of dementia. It is one of the blessings.

So, learn everything real about dementia, and then pay close attention to the one you care for. In your journal, note specific effects of different elements of daily life. This will help you understand how to manage both your lives better. For example, if you see that your mother gets agitated if pushed to hurry, you'll know to leave plenty of time to get ready for a doctor's appointment. If she becomes very sensitive to rain or wind, as many elders with dementia do, you'll know to avoid taking her out in such conditions, if possible. This way, you'll avoid exhausting struggles.

You, and you alone, are the real on-the-spot expert on the person you care for. You are the one who can sense when something has changed. You are the one who knows what makes that person comfortable or uncomfortable. Be prepared to stand up for what you know when necessary. That means you stand up to doctors, to social workers, to siblings, to everyone who assumes they know more about your person than you do. No one is as expert on your person as you are.

What Alzheimer's Looks Like

The Invisible Phase

This is my term for that period of months or years when only the person afflicted is aware that something is wrong with their memory and thinking processes. No one outside this person has any idea of their inner struggle, unless they talk about it – and most people don't. The stress and difficulty of this time of isolation and fear may show outwardly in any of the following ways:

- Emotional changes – becoming depressed, outbursts of anger in someone previously even-tempered, accusations, fearfulness

- Habit changes – not interested in former hobbies, reluctant to socialize, begins drinking heavily

- Changes in appearance – unkemptness, poor choice of clothes, doesn't seem to care about appearance, looks less organized

- Problems at work – no longer carries out duties well, can't follow through on projects, falling standards, inability to manage

- Cognitive problems – can't seem to follow a rational discussion, can't grasp a concept, can't balance a checkbook, can't organize medications

- Memory issues – which may be concealed from others

This is often a very secretive phase where trust issues are paramount. The person doesn't want anyone else to know there's something wrong, often because it is hard to understand what exactly is going on. Nothing feels right, mentally or emotionally. I suspect this phase can go on for years before the issues become outwardly visible as what is usually called the early stage.

The Early Stage

This is dementia as it first looks to outsiders and covers a range of problems. The visible early phase sees an intensification of all the memory, functional, and social issues, which become increasingly stressful for the individual trying to deal with them at the same time that the ability to do so is declining.

This is the point at which family members begin to be concerned. They see that Mother looks less clean, neat, and well dressed, that her hair is no longer so well looked after, that some of her behaviors are odd. She puts salt into her coffee instead of sugar and yet drinks it down without apparent response.

Normal household tasks get ignored and left undone, or are done incompletely, inefficiently, or oddly. Nothing seems to be proceeding smoothly any more. Emotional outbursts may continue. Accusations may be made, against neighbors, family members, bank tellers. Everything is someone else's fault.

Shopping, eating, and driving may all be being done poorly. The refrigerator is full of ice cream but not much food. The stove isn't used for cooking. Family members begin to question if something is wrong and whether they should intervene. Both answers are YES.

Disruption of daily life continues – pots are left to burn on the stove, sleep habits change, things are put away in strange places or lost indefinitely, car accidents happen, or people get lost while driving in familiar territory. This whole period of time, which might be a couple of years, has everyone feeling uneasy, unsettled, and unable to decide what to do. This is when the first family council should take place.

Re-Learning the Person with Dementia

People with dementia change. That is inevitable. Exactly how a person changes is almost totally individual and this is another learning task for you. Note those changes so you can make allowances for them and plan around them.

For example, people who used to be very outgoing and gregarious no longer seem to want to go out. When you try to make them, they seem to withdraw in the crowd. We can guess – and guessing is a very valid part of observation, by the way – that because these people can no longer process information and deal with social contact successfully, the old sense of enjoyment has gone. Instead, they feel alone, fearful, and incapable in a social scene.Caregivers deal with this in different ways. Some will still try to make their person social, thinking that this helps retain abilities.

It is a valid point of view, although not one that I share. Usually people with dementia need less stressful lives in which they are not forced to confront their growing inadequacies. As a caregiver, you are free to make your own care plans for the person you look after. Just don't think you can hold back the disease, because you can't. People often tend to lose interest in what they once cared about and I'm not sure we can, or even should, do much about that.

Although people would like to think it's really true that you can retrain a brain affected by dementia, there is no real proof of this. After all, Nobel prizewinners have Alzheimer's. Observers can easily confuse the pleasure of getting attention with joy in the activity. My observations are that people can be distressed by mental exercises that are too complex. I've seen people slap themselves or beat on their own heads when tormented to carry out intellectual or, even worse, memory tasks. I don't support it.

Maybe, instead, we caregivers need to help them find new rewards. There are many other kinds of satisfaction and amusement available to people with dementia. Perhaps we should look at activities based upon the non-intellectual – creativity, painting, gardening, pets, music. Learn to pick up on any cue that this person mentions from their own life.

Better to learn what works for this person now so you can replace losses with other kinds of reward. The brain has now changed and, with it, the personality. We usually can't move people back to being who they were once they are no longer that same person. We may be able to evoke their former being from time to time, but we can't force it.

Instead, our task is to find that which more suitably meets their needs and helps them to be happy. Many people with dementia become much more at home in their own hearts and may become more emotionally open and available. That openness and availability is where we should try to evoke responses. If we insist on holding onto who this person once was, everyone is left lonely and bereft. This is a center of crisis for many caregivers.

The increasing emotional openness of the person with dementia can be a profound challenge to family members who were more comfortable with reticence and avoidance. It is, however, their own chance to become more emotionally open and available to themselves. It can also be one of the great and curious gifts which dementia has to offer caregivers, if they have the courage to accept it.

Be Prepared

You never know what's going to happen, so be prepared with your care package of necessary information on the person you look after. This should include their Medicare card, any other medical insurance information, social security card, list of current medications, list of current medical conditions, copy of Power of Attorney for Healthcare, copy of Advanced Medical Directives, personal doctor's name and telephone number, and any other relevant papers.

Never give these to anyone and never leave them with anyone. If someone wants to copy down the information, at the hospital admissions desk, for example, stand there and wait for the papers to be returned to you. Hospitals can easily lose your paperwork if you give them a chance. Have a spare copy of the medications list so you can allow an ambulance crew to take them to the hospital if they are answering a 911 call at your house. Put everything in a folder that fits into an easy-grab plastic bag and keep it by the telephone. That way, in an emergency, you can grab and go. Remember to keep everything updated.

If you think that one day you might choose to place your elder in long-term care, do your homework well in advance. Visit likely places in your area so you know what they look and feel like. Note down any that you like the look of and check out their latest state inspection report, which by law they are mandated to keep available for reference for any visitor or official. When you get home, go online and look up their state licensing and check past reports and any citations they've received, since this will help you in your assessment. Small geographical issues – slow flowing water from a washbasin – are not important, but issues of abuse, neglect, and poor care conditions are very important.

Caregiver Toolkit

Usually in Alzheimer's and similar dementias, the emergencies for caregivers are internal – that is, how bad you feel, how angry, how agitated, how sad, and so on. So this is a simple start-up toolkit for you, to help you through the moments and hours when things seem too overwhelming. Do *not* disregard the usefulness of such tools because they look too simple. Caregivers usually tell themselves a *very big lie*, which makes self-help almost impossible. They internally tell themselves that the way they feel now cannot be healed or helped until the problem is over. They then have a sense of personal hopelessness and the guilt of thinking they are wishing for the death of the person they care for.

We need help when we need it. In every moment you can choose to change yourself. You can pick calmness instead of agitation, love instead of anger, breathing instead of tensing. There are a number of extremely simple ways to de-stress the moment and that de-stressing is the key to your peace of mind. You can indeed solve your particular internal problem, the stress you feel, in every moment. You have power to make that choice at any time. So, discipline yourself to make that choice instead of choosing to perpetuate your stress.

The reason so many don't do this is because they are addicted to stress. Addiction to stress is like any other addiction. No one in the caregiving world ever talks about this, but caregivers quickly get addicted to stress because it brings instant energy, albeit long-term harm. The energy of stress is a free drug with terrible side effects.

I'm not denying that caregiver life is genuinely stressful, but Alzheimer's caregivers have been notably unwilling to learn better coping skills. Everyone working with them notices this and wonders about it. I have come to the conclusion that it is the addiction to stress that feeds this reluctance. And this addiction probably has a great deal to do with the fact that many caregivers die before the person they are caring for. So here are five de-stressors:

1. Breathe

Sit down and take ten deep breaths, slowly in and slowly out. Each breath should go all the way from your nose down to below your naval, moving your belly in and out each time. Do this regularly throughout a stressful day. Notice how very shallow and tight your breathing is when you are stressed. This starves your body of oxygen and makes you feel worse and do worse. Using this tool can profoundly change your moments.

Don't believe me? Try it and see. Breath is your lifeline. When stressed, we take in too little air, too seldom. This is a great gift you can give yourself in any moment.

2. Walk away

If the person you care for has become agitated or angry or is just plain driving you crazy in that moment, turn around and walk away. Sit in the garden, lie on the sofa, run a hot bath, pick up a book, play the saxophone – anything that shows you that you are in control of the boundary of your life in this moment.

Even if you have to stay in the same room, you can give yourself the gift of doing something you want to do instead of something you don't. You can mentally walk away. A bonus from this is that the other person often calms down in response to your calm.

3. Don't argue

You can never win an argument with a person who has dementia. Do you know why? Because they have dementia! They are injured irrevocably in their cognitive ability to make sensible arguments. So save your breath. Breathe for yourself instead; then walk away so you can think about why you're trying to force your opinion on a person with dementia. Usually it is because you are angry, which they pick up and return as stubborn resistance.

4. Be absurd

Sometimes our own zaniness is what keeps us caregivers sane, so be absurd. Waltz the cat, bark at the dog, dance around the house. On the whole, people with dementia do not have a whole lot of judgment about our silliness, and that can be very freeing. Try it and enjoy it.

5. Apologize

Let's suppose you lose your cool and express anger at or about the person you are caregiving. A few minutes later, it is very likely that this person will have totally forgotten. That is the time to apologize honestly.

For example: "I'm really sorry I got mad at you. I shouldn't have done that. I just didn't get enough sleep, and blah, blah, blah."

It is very usual for the person with dementia to say, "Oh no, you never lose your temper," or something gratifying like that, because these incidents are not stored in their long-term memory. You get let off the hook for bad behavior and, even better, you are often absolved totally by this person you look after. So next time you lose it, say you're sorry and see what happens. In the immediate moment, you'll feel better for apologizing and, in the long-term, it is rather like absolution – a great comfort. It's one of those quirky little bonuses of caring for people with Alzheimer's. So, enjoy!

Five short problem-solvers – can they really work? You'll have to try them to see for yourself, but here's the reason they often work. When we feel that some aspect of caregiving is a constant, on-going, unbearable, problematic issue, we become stuck in our position. Once we get stuck, we find it impossible to unstick ourselves and it becomes a vicious circle. Doing any of these five things breaks the cycle. Once we break the cycle, everything can change for the better.

A LIFE IN ALZHEIMER'S LAND

I had been told that she had no short-term memory but that did not mean much to me until I saw how it affected Hannah. Every time I left the room, even for a moment or two, she would greet me afresh each time I returned.

"Oh how nice!" she would say, "I'm so happy to see you."

She did not remember I had been sitting next to her a few moments before, talking with her. I enjoyed the warmth and friendliness of these greetings, of which there must have been more than a dozen on my first afternoon with Hannah. I thought it was delightful. I especially enjoyed it when she said, "I shall never forget you!"

Hannah was a big-boned woman with silvery-white hair, a patrician profile that must have taken years to grow into, and a ready smile.

It was easy to feel affection for her right from the start. Like many others who have lived in extremity, I am drawn to those who survive life on the edge and do it well. There could be no doubt that Hannah was living on the very edges of her intellect and yet she seemed very full emotionally.

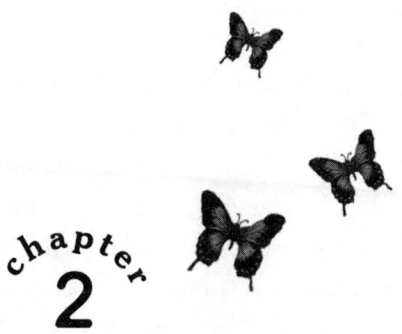

Looking After Number One

If you're going to be a caregiver, it's essential to look after yourself properly. Becoming a caregiver needs as much planning and practice as preparing for the New York Marathon. In fact, being a caregiver is a kind of marathon. You'll be out there and running from the beginning. Don't be deceived into thinking that looking after an old person with dementia will be a slow business.

That person may be slow at walking, eating, reading, and thinking, but your life won't be. From the first day, you'll be multi-tasking and every day will bring a fresh surprise, not always a welcome one. Typically, caregivers stumble into the caregiving life and continue that way, even for years. It's as if people somehow imagine that they really can do this by making it up from day to day. However, that approach is the sure way to exhaustion and depression. I already know you're sensible, or you wouldn't be reading this book, so let's make a sensible plan for healthy caregiving.

We have not, as a society, required this of family caregivers. We have not let people know that there are standards that we expect. That's why right now so many elders are being cruelly looked after by enraged and incapable spouses who will neither let them go where they can get good care nor have the willingness to learn the job properly. Some of this is due to extreme age, of course. We also have a prevailing societal attitude that caregiving doesn't count for much, so there's no real need to have standards for it. Few organizations teach Caregiving 101 to family members, and support groups go only so far.

You, on the other hand, want more, and you want it for yourself and for the person you care for. You want to do this well and you want to survive it well. Right? Right!

The only way to change is to start by changing yourself, and that means, from the beginning, make a plan to care for yourself well. The biggest mistake caregivers make is to ignore what they need. They say things like, "I don't have time to think of myself," or "I'm too tired to do that," or – worst of all – "I don't need help yet."

Wrong! All caregivers need help from day one – or even before day one. There is no such thing as "not needing help yet." The person who says that is already heading into big trouble, so we'll agree right now that it isn't going to be you, is it? You probably know the saying, "It takes a village to raise a child." Well, it also takes a village to care for an elder.

We human beings are tribal people. We have always lived in groups and our survival has always depended upon it. That is because living as a group provides the necessary help and support to make life viable and rewarding. The Dalai Lama describes our most sacred way of human living as "interdependence." That is certainly the only way to successfully live life to its fullest as an elder.

These days, thank goodness, we understand the wrongness of the independence school of thinking. We know it as denial and we recognize it as dysfunctional behavior. We know better now. Not everyone does better yet, but most of us now know better.

What your elderly parents or grandparents might have done, in the way of denial or dysfunction, came out of the generational thought processes of their time. They were raised on a romantic pioneer myth. Everyone was supposed to be independent, never take family troubles outside the family, and never ask for help. They meant well, but they made myths that have become poisonous. When it comes to the lives of elders today, it has become a horribly destructive myth, leaving elderly caregivers tottering while family members don't know how to step in.

Elders who cling to the myth of independence end up living in long-term care situations because of this philosophy. As someone who has worked in elder care and long-term care for almost two decades, I can assure you that it is not people's health conditions that bring them into such care. It is because their support systems have failed.

Everyone who lives long enough gets old. Getting old enough probably means having some difficult health issues to deal with, but most of them can be dealt with equally well at home. What makes the difference? Lack of support systems. Maybe they are the last of their family. More likely their family is not willing or able to care for them because of some past history or just the demands of geographical distance.

It can even happen through a kind of spiritual pride – not wanting their family members to know they were getting old, becoming less able to manage, and being unwilling to ask for needed help. Either way, it's a guaranteed ticket to disaster.

So, as the newest family caregiver, don't you buy that ticket. Take everything we've learned from the self-help, self-improvement, and 12-Step movements, and build a support system so that you can undertake the task of being a caregiver without guaranteed failure.

All caregiving can be hard work sometimes. All family members can be difficult sometimes. These factors are increased exponentially when Alzheimer's or a similar dementia enters the picture. When a person has dementia, you can't count on their memory and you can't count on the rational to shape their life normally. You never know what that person might get up to. It's one of the things I've always liked about people with dementia, but it can also be stressful.

Being a caregiver to a family member is at least three times the work it would be for an outsider. Past history and the family psyche at work, with all its inheritance and emotional debt, can pile on intensity. Additionally, when caregiving is given in the context of an illness from which this person cannot recover, it is a foreshadowing of loss, pain, and personal dread. For some caregivers, grief may weigh down the process from the beginning.

Caregiving is never only a practical matter. It is a relationship of exchange and struggle. It contains multiple issues for both parties – issues of feelings and mutual history – that may pile on top of already arduous and demanding tasks. It is seldom routinely easy, not even for professional strangers skilled and practiced at what they do. Between family members of equal status, it can be a hard relationship to develop.

As a nurse once said in one of my support groups, "I'm a nurse – I should know all this. And I do. But this is my mother and it's all so much harder than I imagined it would be."

Learning a task is one thing. Applying that to your own relative, especially your parent, is more challenging. That's natural, especially at first. However, it is important never to listen to those people who insist that being an Alzheimer's caregiver is a depressing, impossible task. That's just not true and there is a potent history behind that myth.

Alzheimer's disease was first named in 1910, but was not popularly spoken of until 1969, when the term senile dementia began to be dropped in favor of the name Alzheimer's disease. The first generation of people who discovered they were dealing with Alzheimer's, from 1960 onwards, had very little help. They did their best in a world where almost no one understood the issues. These pioneers tended to be the spouses of men and women with dementia, often already in their own seventies or older.

They often did not have an understanding of dementia, or the tools to help them manage well, or access to such tools. They did not have the habit of sharing their emotional passages with outsiders, or perhaps even with themselves. They were almost alone in a situation which one person alone cannot manage. Unfortunately, out of their sense of bewildered isolation and loss, a picture of dementia and Alzheimer's was created which still dominates our societal view to this day.

It has afflicted caregiving for nearly forty years and it's time to challenge it. I say this, not to criticize, but to point out that it is now our blessing to have all the self-help tools from the 12-Step programs and personal growth movements, and the easy availability of therapy and counseling. We also know that on-going problems require on-going support and guidance. We are also more familiar with the whole idea of Alzheimer's, even if we don't know its nuances. So you come to caregiving at a fortunate time.

It is absolutely vital that you bring all those helpful tools into your life as a caregiver. You need help, support, and training, so take responsibility for getting those things. You can't do it alone and you need to meet and accept the challenges of the journey as well-armed as possible. Do not be like so many other dementia caregivers who resist the acquisition of skills and won't ask for help. Don't take on that kind of addiction to stress that afflicts caregivers. We have been reluctant to challenge the issue, but now we must. The price that stress-addicted caregivers pay is so heavy. Stress itself is the gateway to all our major illnesses.

That's not a vague theory. About sixty-six percent of older caregivers die on the job. Among younger family members, who may have brought a parent home to be cared for, family life can be devoured by the caregiving of an elder. This is not anyone's fault, but comes down to both sides being unwilling or unable to tackle boundary and care issues in a straightforward, practical way. Ironically, it is the family relationship itself that makes that so hard.

So, you can probably see how there are actually two equally important issues in caregiving. One is how you will take care of your family member, and the other is how you will take care of your own life and nurture the things that bring you vitality, joy, and transcendence.

Stress Marks

Stress can infiltrate your own being without you really knowing it. We all think we know how we feel when we're stressed because each of us probably has some major indicator that we are familiar with. We are anxious, have digestive upsets, can't sleep, and have other symptoms. However, stress can manifest in many more ways that we often don't recognize, so here's a handy checklist:

Physical Symptoms

- Aches and pains around the body that may settle in one obvious place – your shoulder or your back – or may migrate about, so that every day you have a different ache

- Muscle tension and stiffness

- Problems in your elimination system, such as diarrhea or constipation

- Nausea or dizziness without any apparent cause
- Sleep problems
- Heart pains or rapid heartbeat, without medical cause
- Weight gain or loss
- Skin problems
- Frequent colds, infections, or allergy outbreaks
- Loss of libido

Psychological Symptoms

- Short-term memory problems affect anyone of any age when life is stressful
- Inability to make decisions
- Negative outlook
- Poor concentration
- Lack of mental clarity
- Anxiety
- Fretfulness
- Lack of proportion
- Fearfulness
- Mood swings
- Inability to sit still
- Inability to relax
- Easily angered
- Tenseness and irritability
- Loneliness
- Depression
- Feeling overwhelmed

Behavioral Symptoms

- Binge eating
- Sleep changes
- Use of alcohol or drugs to mitigate stress
- Over-reaction to others
- Procrastination
- Self-isolation and avoidance of others

HALT

This is a self-help device from the 12-Step movement, but it is a wonderful short checklist for knowing that you need immediate intervention *by* you *for* you. At any time when you feel you have really lost it, run the HALT check and apply the necessary short-term self-rescue. Are you *Hungry, Angry, Lonely, or Tired*?

You can apply the antidote for any of these. This acronym also reminds you what components your support system needs. Hungry means you need to eat something, of course. Angry means you need to go out and instantly defuse that anger a little. Here's my favorite instant fix for anger at a person. Write that person's name on a piece of paper, go into a room where you have privacy, and then jump up and down on it. It's an absurd piece of theater that lowers the anger pressure and also makes me laugh at my own silliness, which further takes off the pressure.

Tired means you need to take a break. The great thing about people with dementia is that they are pretty accepting of anything you do. You can lie down on the sofa and snooze in their presence. You can go sit up close, lean against them, and fall asleep. That way, you know where they are and if they move, you'll wake up again.

The bigger challenge is in the word *lonely*. Being a caregiver can be very lonely sometimes. You need a support system. Oh, did I say that three thousand times already? If you don't have a friend, relative, pastor, or dementia phone-buddy, then call the various support hotlines. Before you even begin caregiving, start making that all-important list of people to call when you would like company – what my friend Nancy calls "the 3 a.m. phone-call list." She says she has never actually called any of them at 3 a.m., but she feels much better knowing that she could.

Sometimes, you can help your lonely self by taking the person you care for out to eat. There will be others around and sometimes this can be enough to help you feel less lonely.

Instead of just letting yourself be washed over by a great tide of caregiving toxin, make a list. Actually, make two lists. On one, write down the major problems in your caregiving life right now. On the other, write down what would help you right now. Then take a good long look at your caregiving problems and start planning what to do about them. Almost every problem on the caregiving list would probably involve getting help.

Help!

Isn't it interesting that the same word *help* can be used to deal with both sides of caregiving? When overwhelmed, confused, and lost in tasks of helping others, we want to yell "HELP!" And no wonder, because we might occasionally feel we are living in an on-going emergency lifestyle that has no end.

The solution is getting help, again with two meanings – help as knowledge and necessary skills, and help in the shape of a person to assist you. There are times when all of us need both kinds of help and, as a caregiver, it is essential that you don't think you are supposed to do everything yourself.

If the elder you care for has money, use it to pay for extra help or extra services. There is absolutely no point in saving their money when it needs to be used for their quality of life. It is a good investment to give money in exchange for good services that enable you to become a better caregiver. If you have money, do the same. If neither of you have money, start figuring out how you're going to get that help. Call your local senior services and every possible volunteer help agency as well as any church or spiritual community you can track down and ask, ask, ASK!

Support Groups

You are going to need a support group. Fortunately, the American

Alzheimer's Association has them all over the United States, and in Canada there is the Alzheimer Society of Canada. There will be at least one within reach of you wherever you live, and often there may be several. Most towns and cities also have other caregiver support groups. Sometimes care facilities have them; sometimes a church will be hosting one. Your local Area Agency on Aging will have a list of local resources that they'll send you. And of course, there is the wonderful Internet with its information resources, chat rooms, forums, and helpful websites. (For more information, see Resources)

Please plan from the very beginning to go to a support group. Don't leave it until you're totally stressed out. Don't tell yourself, "It'll be a bunch of people just complaining about stuff – I don't need that." That's a very retro idea about support groups that people use to persuade themselves not to go. Not getting support is a very bad idea. It is dysfunctional, and Alzheimer's caregivers really don't need any extra dysfunction in their lives. They already have enough to power a small city with frustration. In fact, even before you start being a caregiver, if you haven't already, go to a support group meeting or two anyway. You'll really appreciate its existence.

Learn Alzheimer's

Save yourself from useless frustration, stress, anger, and bewilderment by learning all you can about Alzheimer's. That way you won't waste time trying to re-train a person, blaming a person for their disease, or expecting unrealistic results from what you do, say, or want. There is an entire chapter later on understanding Alzheimer's, but here I'm just reminding you that you need to learn what typical Alzheimer's may look like. That knowledge will help you.

Those with Alzheimer's are not as crazy as society tells us. People are not really empty, absent, and gone away. The strange things they do are usually a way of trying to communicate, coming from a person whose skills have been stolen by a disease.

If you know how to listen, people with dementia make more sense than you might think.

Remember that Alzheimer's is not a mental illness, but a physical brain problem. Due to brain changes, the usual reliable pathways of thinking become blocked. Some areas of the brain are especially vulnerable to this, the parts where memory functions, for example. What is happening in Alzheimer's is that the person can no longer access these functions very easily, so they try hard to make sense of things, to construct memory that works, and to live in a world becoming increasingly full of bewilderment.

This person is not imagining that space aliens have taken over their naval. This is not a brain filled with hallucinatory fantasies and paranoid scenarios. This is not a psychosis, paranoid schizophrenia, or bipolar condition. It is a physically failing brain function.

That does not exclude the possibility that a few people have what is usually referred to as a dual-diagnosis. That is, they do have both a mental illness *and* Alzheimer's or some similar dementia. And, by the way, you may also find someone being referred to as having Alzheimer's when in fact they probably have a lifelong, undiagnosed mental illness. So, it is not surprising that people can still be confused by what these terms mean. That is why it is important to learn what typical Alzheimer's may look like.

Preparations for Caregiving

Learn thyself!

While you may well know yourself as you are, you don't know yourself as a caregiver until you start being a caregiver. You can assume that anything difficult now will be magnified once you're a caregiver. If you are someone who is easily made anxious or finds it hard to sleep under stress, assume these may become significant factors in your caregiving life.

Include deliberate stress management techniques and practice them every day. If you are easily stressed, I already know you don't want to do that because people who live with stress typically choose not to deal with it. Since nagging you won't help, instead turn the question around in a different way. Would *you* want to be looked after by you if you were anxious and sleep-starved? Ah hah! That's why you need to find ways to deal with stress, including some kind of regular exercise – just plain walking is one of the best stress management tools – and habits that lead to relaxation.

The music you like, books you like, activities you like – these can all help. If you anger easily, you are definitely going to have to find ways to deal with that. Anger management courses are great for people like you. Failing that, at least be willing to read books and listen to CD courses about anger which will give you better self-management tools. Failing that, practice counting to ten.

Whatever your bad habits are, they will intensify under caregiving, so you must plan accordingly by safeguarding yourself where you are weak. If you eat through stress, you must be very careful to plan and buy the right kinds of food to prevent that. So many care workers are obese because that is how they deal with the stress and the loneliness of their work. Don't stock your fridge with stress-binge foods. Just don't have them there at all. Instead, get those other foods you know you should eat, but don't. Read self-help books from your library, buy them from amazon.com online, or borrow from your friends.

Last of all, have fun with this! Don't think you can't. I've been a caregiver for nearly twenty years and there's a secret you need to know. There can be a lot of fun, happiness, and amusement in the typical Alzheimer's day, so go for it.

Hobbies

If you never had hobbies before, you'd better invent some for your caregiving life. Have books to read and movies to watch. Now is the time to begin your new hobby of clock repair or drawing or writing, because you will probably have time for those things.

Take an entertainment kit to work with you, with some ambitious projects too, as long as they fit into your bag, your room, and your caregiving life. If you always meant to grow your own sprouts, learn to cook, or study a foreign language, now's the time.

Maybe you always wanted to play the piano. Well, buy a keyboard and a pair of headphones and there you go. Get yourself a laptop, if you don't already have one, and do an online study course. It's not that you will have endless hours for these things – some days maybe you won't have even one. It's that things that matter to you – dreams you have, good intentions you'd like to fulfill – are going to help you survive the work and commitment ahead.

You and what you value and dream about are as important as the work that you do. When you value and feed your own inner being, you increasingly become the person who can pretty much deal with anything, especially with yourself.

A LIFE IN ALZHEIMER'S LAND

My first weeks with Hannah were spent getting to understand what parts of her intellect were still functional. This was a woman who had gone to university at the age of sixty-four to earn her degree. She had lived in Berkeley for fifteen years, had gone to the Pacific Films Archives in the university almost every evening to see foreign films, had been a staunch volunteer at the Berkeley Free Clinic and a very active member of the synagogue, and had walked two hours in the Berkeley Hills every day. Her life had been rich and significant.

Now she had become a woman who could not remember to use toilet paper unless cued to do so. She no longer connected nouns with their actual form in the world. She could not pick out a knife and a fork by name. She did not know and could not remember our names. At first, I felt a little sad about this, and then I noticed something. She would come close to me and peer into my face, and then light dawned.

"Ah!" she cried delightedly. "It's you! I'm so glad!"

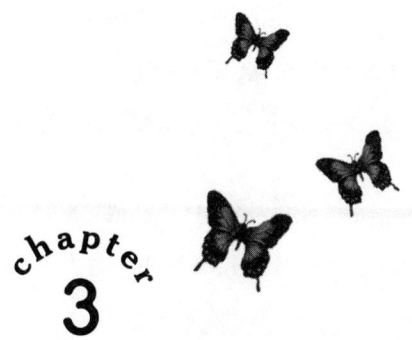

Who's the Boss?
You Are!

Well, you're the boss of some people anyway. If you're a family caregiver with siblings, then you and the sibs have to come to an agreement about who's boss. This probably means a call for a family council.

Most people never think of doing this. They just struggle haphazardly through the months and years. Don't let this be you. Have a council, ask for what you need, and see if you can get it. If people do not step up to the plate, at least you know where you stand. Stop counting on them and start getting help elsewhere. And you must. Dealing with dementia is *not* a one-person job. You will only end up exhausted, possibly ill, and certainly no longer nice to know. So, onto the family council in which you ask for what is needed.

Get everyone together, preferably in the same location or, second choice, at least all on the computer or via telephone, for a serious discussion and decision-making conference. It can be useful to send out a list of the possible issues before this council.

To do this discussion well, some rules are required, whether they are tacit or everyone is required to agree to them in advance. Before you laugh and say, "My family would never do that..." just remember that probably no one ever asked them to do things in a grown-up way instead of continuing their usual routines. The rules for family negotiation are:

- No recriminations about the past
- No advance accusations about the future, as in "You never…"
- Stay in the present moment and work on the plan
- Respect differences and use the individual strengths of each family member
- Negotiate to make a more-or-less consensual agreement
- Have a list of issues, which can be added to or changed
- Be as brief as possible
- Do not to finish without a plan, even if you have to agree to further discussion

These are issues you have to decide on:

1. Who's in charge of finances?

Even if that is decided to be a non-caregiver, daily finances must be clearly established and available for the on-the-spot caregiver. An actual budgeted amount of money may take more than one meeting to determine. Be ready with a detailed list of average daily, weekly, and monthly totals. This is very important because a squabbling family will definitely squabble about money, and ugly accusations can so easily be made. True or false as these may be, they will dishearten you from the task of caregiving.

2. Who's in charge of health care decision-making?

This is usually taken care of by appointing one of the family members to have medical power of attorney. Be clear about who will speak on behalf of the parent, and honor the parent's wishes as expressed in a living will or medical directive. Determine whether everyone agrees to honor these wishes. In these times, even if a parent has dementia it is still usually legally accepted that this person is clear about his or her wishes in the case of serious or life-threatening conditions. Copies of all empowering documents should be lodged with your parent's doctor and possibly with the local hospital (although they can lose documents), and it's smart to keep copies on hand.

The family needs to talk about the role of the daily caregiver in decision-making in the case of an emergency. When this happens, the holder of the medical power of attorney may not be immediately available and medical help may be immediately needed.

The family needs to agree on acceptable actions on the part of the caregiver and be ready to back them. Some major decisions need to be made, such as the decision to resuscitate or not, and these need to be backed by documentation, such as a DNR (Do Not Resuscitate) sheet. Most doctors and local hospitals have these, and your parent's doctor is the one who will go through this with your parent at the next doctor visit.

These are not trivial issues. If you ordinarily have problems with your siblings, imagine standing around your parent's hospital bed quarreling and swapping accusations about who is trying to murder Mom or Dad. Believe me, it happens, and it can cause family rifts that are never repaired.

When siblings have love and attention issues from the past that they have not dealt with, relative to a seriously ill parent, some may want to keep them alive indefinitely because of these unsettled emotional issues. It is the last chance, as it were, to grab that attention. Sometimes siblings may even kidnap an old and frail parent from each other as part of that same issue. It is an ugly situation unlikely ever to be healed after the death of that parent – hence, the need for family council and signed legal documents for difficult decisions.

You can get these forms from a variety of sources, most of them free. You can buy them in stationery stores or online, some are available at hospitals or from your doctor, and some may possibly be found in your local library. Nolo Press of Berkeley, California, publishes legal books for ordinary folks with useful forms already provided.

For simple decisions – whose name goes on the parent's bank account, what the advanced medical directives are, or signing a DNR order – most families do not go to a lawyer.

However, if your family is prone to dissension and accusation, you might want to make sure everything is signed and sealed. You know them, you choose. If you have no siblings at all, it can simplify life a great deal, as well as complicate it in other ways.

3. Who's in charge of the daily routine?

This has to be the hands-on caregiver and all family members have to agree to allow that. Sometimes, family members become fanatical about the health regimes of their elders and take the opportunity of their frailty as a chance to clean them up at last.

Enforced vegetarianism, fanatical food policing, new exercise routines, interference with medications – all bad, probably. Nutritional renewal of an elder in ill health, with dementia? It's probably not going to happen and may cause a lot of distress, certainly emotional and possibly even digestive. Continue to accept a parent's likes and dislikes and, by all means, step up food quality as consistent with kindness. Accept that your likes will probably not be theirs. Nothing divides generations as much as food and cooking.

For example, I've found that many Caucasian elders over eighty have a standard list of what they don't like, for example, strong coffee, whole wheat bread, shrimp, mushrooms, garlic and spices, and exotic fruits and vegetables. I think of that as the Heartland diet. You can't make them enjoy Starbucks and mangoes if they don't. Leave it alone. Cook what they want to eat – then they'll eat it. And that's a good contribution to their overall health. Good food is best, but uneaten food doesn't help anyone. Understand it is probably too late to bring about major health changes at a late age and, by the way, late introduction of low-fat, no-salt, no-sugar diets usually only curtails the appetite.

There is almost no medical research that backs up the usefulness of such late-in-life changes. Most elders need color, taste, and a combination of variety and the familiar on one plate to engage their appetites.

The only really useful change is the introduction of additional enzymes to aid digestion, since most elders have a serious reduction in the natural digestive enzymes, probably due to age and effects of medication. More on this subject will be found in later chapters.

For exercise, try to find something they might try. Chair yoga for elders, for example, is easy to do and has definite benefits. Tai Chi modified, likewise. However, if your parent does not want to do these things, let it go. You probably can't make them healthy and there's no point in making them miserable.

4. Who's in charge of your parent – your parent or you?

This is the decision that causes the most distress to well-meaning children. Good children want to respect their elders. They don't want to trespass on their freedoms. They don't want to make them do things for their own good. They don't want to forcibly change the life of their parents. And these are good attitudes.

Yet I am constantly amazed at the ways in which people feel they have a right to boss their elders about concerning things that have nothing to do with health or safety. Many people are plainly mistaken about what constitutes self-endangering behavior. Too often, endangering behavior is simply a version of "I don't like you doing that, so therefore it's bad for you."

Let me outline what your parent has a normal right to be like, whether you like it or not. It's a little guidance for those people I think of as the Pajama Police – not you, of course. You know, those other people who have somehow confused the end of civilization as we know it with wearing pajamas past noon. Feel free to read this section to your parent, and be sure to pay attention to it for your own management plan of your parent. Here we go:

Ten Things They Can't Make You Do When You're Old

1. They can't make you take a shower. No matter what the Pajama Police think, not taking a shower doesn't hurt you. Even Social Services can't, and won't, make you take a shower. You have a right to not take showers. Cleanliness is not next to godliness. Someone's mother came up with that one. Moreover, being dirty is not bad for your health. If it were, all little boys would be dead. PS: It wouldn't hurt to wash though, especially if you're going to sit next to me.

2. They can't make you buy new underwear. You have a right to wear underwear that's full of holes. You have a right to wear no underwear at all.

3. They can't make you eat your greens and they can't stop you from eating ice-cream – lots of it, all the time. With cookies – lots of them.

4. They can't stop you from wearing pajamas as long as you want to. Actually, with the current changes in fashion, you'll be glad to know

you can wear your pajamas to go shopping and no one will even think, "Why, goodness me, those are his pajamas!" Be sure to leave the bedroom slippers at home though, because they give you away every time.

5. They can't put you in a home because you can't remember things. Not remembering is *not* a sign of dementia. Poor short-term memory is a normal glitch of aging and it doesn't mean you have dementia. Losing yours keys – that's normal. If you can't remember where you put your home, however, now *that* is alarming. Maybe you do have dementia.

6. They can't make you take your pills. You can take or leave your pills. You have a legal right to *not* take pills. Even if you live in a care facility, as a matter of fact, you still have a right to refuse your pills. I'm not saying you should. I'm just saying no one has the right to make you. Not even your doctor. Not even the police. Frankly, given the appalling statistic that over sixty-five percent of all admissions of elders to hospital are due to their medications, not to their illnesses, maybe you just *should* refuse your pills. Well, okay, just take the important ones. The ones without which you fall to the floor, turn blue, go into insulin shock – take those pills. Even though I can't make you.

7. They can't make you go to bed. You can go to bed any time you want to. Or you need never go to bed at all. You can sleep in your chair, in your car (though preferably not while driving), on your sofa, in the garage.

8. They can't make you get up early, or at all, for that matter. Although, if you never get up you'll probably die of some kind of catastrophic health event. The Pajama Police are usually very keen on people getting up early. There is apparently a moral superiority to the act of getting up early enough to milk a herd of cows, even though you don't have any. So the Pajama Police, who always get up early, feel an urgency about making other people get up early. There is absolutely no proof at all that getting up early is healthier, and I know for a fact it doesn't make you wealthier or wiser.

9. They can't make you stay awake. The older most people get, the more they appreciate little naps throughout the day. It's a fact of life. It's

a fact of old age. Doesn't anyone learn from their old cats and their old dogs? As a matter of fact, studies have shown that really smart people are also people who nap. It's good for your creativity. Sleeping is the time when the body repairs itself. Do too little of it and you're in trouble. Thinking, going inward, daydreaming, remembering – these are the true processes of old age. It is the time of once more reviewing life and setting things to right inside your own heart. That is appropriate behavior, often done best while lying in bed.

10. They can't make you move out of your house. Not without taking you to court to prove you're incompetent. Otherwise, they can't make you move. They can bully you, torment you, nag you, but if you really don't want to move, then don't. *But*, you'd better make sure you have the help you need to stay there safely. If you don't, well that's just plain stupid. Sorry, but there it is. It's not tough, strong, independent, or admirable when you don't seek out and accept what you need to remain at home safely. It's just plain dumb and self-destructive. Wake up and smell that coffee burning.

Smart people stay home until they die. They get the help they need. They do what they can to make life work. They accept family help. They accept their meals on wheels. Then, by Jove, they close the door, put on their jammies, eat ice cream and cookies in bed, and then have a good long nap. Ah, now that's the good life for someone on the edge but not over the edge of dementia, or someone just very old. However, there must be exceptions for the sake of safety, health, and well-being.

Once you realize a parent is endangered and no longer able to make their life safe and well-supported, you must take over. When one parent is abusive of the other, you must act. When a parent becomes a resident in the house of an adult child, this changes the in-charge decisions.

Just so you know, I have never known a family to intervene too soon in the life of a parent needing care. Never. By the time a family is discussing this or thinking about it, it is already late. They are thinking and talking about it because of a discernible decline in the parent's quality of life. If a parent no longer eats well, can no longer live alone safely, or cannot manage daily life in such a way that his or her quality of life is supported, then it is time for intervention.

Certain declines may be distressing to the family but not to the elder, such as being more unkempt, wearing grubby clothes, and not showering much. These may be regrettable, but they are not threatening to health and are not reasons to move this person into care against their will.

Instead, if possible, arrange for help to come to this person. Organize help with family members or hire someone to help with washing, grooming, showering, and making meals. Many services are available through local elder services or state health services. Call your local Area Agency on Aging and ask. (See Resources for more information) You will be pointed in the right direction and you might find that VA benefits, Medicare, or state health-care plans apply to the situation. These folks will be using already well-established local care workers.

Families who don't really want to deal with the issues of hiring will say, "We can't find anyone we trust," or "There's no one out there to hire." Actually, there are plenty of good, honest helpers out there to be hired. Finding them takes the same kind of work you might once have put into finding good childcare or babysitting services for your kids or for your pets.

Ask around, advertise, and use due diligence – check references, have an Internet service run a check on your candidate, have a trial period, and take it from there. Never let anyone start working before you've done all of these things. Never.

If someone is so eager to start that they want to be there that day, there's something wrong. It's not good since it shows desperation. Maybe this is a felon or a person with a drug habit. Take the time to do the research. After all, once you've found the right person, this relationship can keep your parent home, safe, and looked-after for years.

Now, supposing your parent refuses to have help at home? Supposing your father says, "I don't need someone coming in – I can manage!" and yet you know he yells at your mom because he's old, ill, and overwhelmed by her dementia needs?

This is where you step up and assert yourself. You must make it clear that this is not an option, that you need to know someone is there helping them. Take it upon yourself to say, "I know you say that, Dad, but

I worry so much about you both…" and so on. The parent who doesn't want help finds it really hard to block the care and input of a determined child – and that's exactly what you're counting on. Manipulation? You bet it is! And a great management tool for stubborn elders it is, too.

When adult children don't stand up to a parent there is usually a history of intimidation. The parent has a history of anger, punitive attitudes, rough speech, and sometimes even violence. I have even seen healthcare professionals fail to stand up to parents like this. When the well-being and care of the other parent is in jeopardy, you have to do something. You can't just give way on this. Bring in all your siblings, an outside social worker, even Adult Protective Services.

"Well, if you won't have someone here, then you're really going to have to move into an assisted living. There aren't any alternatives to this, so why don't you try someone for a bit and see?" you say firmly but kindly.

No guarantees, but this usually works about ninety percent of the time. But I have to tell you I once met an elderly couple in Arizona who had, as they put it, "run away from home" because of just this situation. They were two thousand miles away from home, with no forwarding address, when I met them – and they were very happy. Well, at least their daughter and son-in-law could let go of having to take care of the needs of their elders in that circumstance.

On the whole, when it really comes down to the wire, most people know when something has to change and usually they will go with it. As a ninety-year-old told her niece, after I had been called in to tell that elder that henceforth she would have a live-in caregiver, "I'm not happy about this, not happy at all." Actually, she remained more or less as happy as she had been before. She just had better meals. Most elders, even those with dementia, know that essential changes often have to be made in life. That's the wisdom of living long.

Then there's the elder who is in denial about what he or she needs and consumes in family effort in terms of their care and says, "Well, I do everything for myself. I don't know what your problem is." This person may still be in his or her own home or may actually be living in your home, in the middle of your family life, eating up all its energy like a termite and yet denying it. Don't get into a power struggle. Instead, recognize this for what it is – denial based upon self-deception or fear.

You, in fact, hold all the power in this situation, and you need to be kind or you'll feel awful later. Try saying something like this: "I understand it's hard for you to admit you need help from us, but you do, and we want to make sure you'll get what you need without all of us being exhausted."

Then go forward with your plan, either to get extra help in the house or have your parent move into a different living situation. Whichever happens, your parent will adjust – not always happily, but as happily as that parent's life pattern has been. An habitually resentful person will stay resentful; a usually happy person will return to reasonable happiness.

I have an Alzheimer's web page and people can email me for help, advice, or just input on their situation. One family emailed me saying their Jewish mother had been raised in Brooklyn but now all her surviving friends had moved to Florida. "We wonder whether, if we moved her to a very nice elder apartment complex in Jerusalem, she might be happy there?" they asked.

Now, I didn't know these people at all but I felt that their question had a strong implication in it that somehow their mother was not habitually happy. In my return email, I asked them what their mother's ability to be happy had been so far in her life. If it was high, I said, then perhaps the move would continue to enhance her happiness. I said she would probably be as happy or unhappy as she had been in general. Their mission, I said, should be to find somewhere that was safe and offered good life quality and the chance of agreeable companionship. Happiness, or not, would be up to her, and she would do whatever she usually did.

5. Who's in charge of the doctor – your parent, the doctor, or you?

Of course, the doctor is in charge of medical information and advice. The patient and the patient's representative – that's you – are free to decide what to do about taking that advice. For the sake of optimal health, you have to become well informed about elder care.

You need to be sure that your elder's doctor is suitable for an elder and especially for one with dementia. Gerontology is not well-studied by most doctors today, which tells you a lot about the respect the medical profession has for older people. Old-age is routinely classified as a medical failure and the old person as medically failed. Seek a doctor with interest in and respect for elders, as well as knowledgeable about dementia caregiving and its issues. What you need is someone capable of very straightforward communication and able to negotiate with you over care issues and requirements without feeling defensive.

What's the negotiation about? It's about the fact that old people don't always do well with new medicine, though they might. It's about the fact that, by the time you're eighty-five, you can eat anything you can eat. So, if it doesn't make you sick, then you can eat it. This translates into very limited sugar for a diabetic, but never mind the cholesterol of a ninety-year-old because cholesterol drugs have side effects you don't want arriving in the life of a ninety-year-old.

Drug companies, other than those trying to market Alzheimer drugs, are not much interested in the elderly. They much prefer slightly unwell forty-five-year-olds who could have a good forty years of buying medicine ahead of them. Elders generally are not included in industrial trials of medicines for that reason. The typical drug-study participant is a thirty-five-year-old male. That is probably why the most common reason for hospital admission in people aged sixty-five and over is reaction to medications, especially a new medication.

Dr. Joe Graedon is a Harvard-educated pharmacist and author of many terrific consumer books on drugs and their side effects. He is very concerned about the way consumers and their needs are handled by drug companies and medication development. He recommends that, unless you have a rare illness from which you are about to die, you only use medications that have been on the market for at least three years, and preferably five.

As someone who had a small care-home for elders, I must say our biggest problem was not the basic health conditions of our residents, but changes in medications. We finally had to ask our doctor not to give anything new unless there was an especially necessary reason. And I had to ban that nice doctor — and he was a wonderful doctor for our elders — from kindly handing out free samples given to him by drug company representatives because they always brought troubles. People fell down, developed skin rashes, and so on.

You have to be in charge of this issue. Be willing to insist nicely on policies to protect your elder from unnecessary and possibly harmful medication changes. Be willing to politely point out, if it's true, that your elder is doing okay on the present drug regime and ask the doctor not to fix what doesn't need repair.

This is the gatekeeper's duty and you are the gatekeeper. It doesn't mean you think you're a doctor. It means you think you are your elder's guardian angel – and you are. The wrong new medicine, after all, can cause your elder to fall, break a hip, and never be able to resume normal life again. When you have time, look up every one of your elder's drugs on the Internet for reported side effects. Then compare that with what you notice in their daily life.

You find three drugs that may cause dizziness and your mom is dizzy? Ask your doctor for an opinion on this, and also ask whether there are equally good drugs without that particular side effect. This doesn't offend good doctors. They understand that you are indeed the gatekeeper.

Bad doctors may react negatively and, if they do, just thank that doctor and get a different one. Your elder pays enough money a year on health in old age to buy a small tropical island, going by current Medicare charges, so consumer satisfaction is certainly a serious issue and the safety of an elder even more so.

Nurture a good relationship with your pharmacist because pharmacists never feel defensive about medications. After all, they didn't prescribe them. Therefore, they are ready to willingly share what they know and what they have observed in their customers. We had great help and guidance from our pharmacist, and on at least one occasion they probably saved the life of one resident by urging me to take her to the emergency room immediately.

6. Who's in charge of social life?

You. Most frail or health-challenged elders don't necessarily feel up to a wild social life. A person with dementia will often begin to avoid it altogether and you probably can't usefully make them start all over again. If they begin to avoid social interactions, it's because they are afraid and feeling inadequate.

It becomes hard to follow a group conversation and put it all together logically. Being around too many people increases feelings of threat and confusion. Far from being a comfort, social stuff becomes scary and just too demanding. Consider one-on-one visits with a friend of your parent. Think about getting a pet for someone isolated by dementia. Even people who never liked pets before may adapt well to one after their illness develops. If you do this, adopt an older pet from a shelter. Usually these have had older owners who died and other people don't want to adopt a portly old dog. Yet these dogs and cats know the routine very well.

They are slow, comfortable with quiet routines, and often very well-adapted to the physical issues of elders. They are often very good at knowing when something is wrong and are very likely to come get you if necessary. They are also a great buffer against the terrible loneliness of losing your life while you actually are still living it. They don't impinge on the memories issues; they are satisfied with their owner in the present moment. This is often more than their owner's family might be. So think of this pet as your sibling helper, too.

If you and the sibs decide on a family Thanksgiving, for example, make sure you assign an attentive, kindly family member to be the *new best friend* of your parent. That way, your elder won't suffer the I'm-all-alone-in-a-crowd abandonment, which you'll see whenever you watch an elder with dementia in the midst of a family circle. The kindly family member will be Mommy for the day, that person who watches out for and reassures them, and knows when a little nap is needed.

This is not to talk down about dementia, by the way. I don't think old people with dementia are children. I think they are elders with rich, full, and difficult years whose coping skills and brain capacity are struggling at primary levels of being, like a child's.

I think some of the ways of managing an elder with dementia who is in difficulty draw upon the same types of skills that a parent uses with a child. I use that term in order to remind us all, including my own impatient self, to slow down, talk softly, speak simply, and be a warm, supportive presence in order to calm the almost constant fear that otherwise overwhelms those with dementia in challenging situations.

You Are the Boss of Your Heart

Much of the difficulty of Alzheimer's comes from the way it tears up our hearts. It is very important that you take your heart and your feelings into your own care. Nurture and apply good commonsense logic to both. This is why. When we make emotional pictures that trouble us, they are simply that – invented pictures. So choose not to do that. Choose to live one day at a time.

Don't project feelings on anyone else. Don't decide that because you, from your non-Alzheimer viewpoint, would hate to have dementia, therefore your mother hates to have it. Actually, very few people with dementia hold onto that idea or feeling for long. From time to time, moment to moment, yes. All the time, no. We project all that onto them just as we turn away from people in wheelchairs because we couldn't bear to be those people. But those people get on with their lives, which are whatever they are as each day unfolds. So, let go of that.

Let go of feeling it is somehow your duty to take on this disease and try to halt its progress. Medical science might do that, but you? No, not likely. It is not your job to exercise your parent's brain so it doesn't decline further. And there's nothing very definite to show that you or anyone else could succeed in that. Just live your life.

Don't heap an imaginary burden of guilt on yourself. Caregiving already has its burdens. Add more and you actually become a worse caregiver. Whatever you feel, whatever you think, whatever you imagine can all be brought under the supportive and kindly discipline of spiritual or anti-stress guidance. You can meditate. You can use discipline to stop obsessive sorrow and guilt-laden thoughts. You can become the boss of you.

The truth is that there can be a lot of satisfaction and happiness in an average Alzheimer's day and that is the place to live. Yes, this stuff is hard and there will be sorrows, but you really don't have to move up onto Lonely Street and book yourself and your mother into the Heartbreak Hotel. Take the deeper, more profound, more deeply spiritual approach, and live your life in the present moment with loving-kindness towards yourself and others.

There are some misleading studies about Alzheimer's which suggest that various feel-good things can prevent it. However, some of the best brains on the planet have Alzheimer's – Nobel prizewinners, great painters, great singers, and great spiritual beings. Nothing right now guarantees our safety from dementia.

There are many things we can do that bring better quality to life, and we should do them. There are many attitudes and spiritualities than can enhance our soul life and we should practice them. We need to live life for its own good, not in fear of an unknown future. So, practice fearless spirituality and loving-kindness. Forgive your own shortcomings. Sleep well. Eat wisely. That's good enough to start with. With that daily exercise, you'll become a great and inspirational caregiver.

A LIFE IN ALZHEIMER'S LAND

This was how it became clear to me that there were different kinds of memory. Her biodata memory – pretty much destroyed. Her sense-of-the-familiar memory – available with variable access. Then I noticed that when I helped her get dressed – without which she might put her socks on her hands – she found it hard at first and then suddenly slipped into an old, well-established body habit which led her successfully through the rest of the process.

So clearly there was also a sense memory which could be accessed. To access these different kinds of memory, Hannah needed time and no stress. Actually, to function at all Hannah needed time and no stress. Relating to people needed time. Talking with her needed time. When people wanted to hurry her, or were in a hurry themselves, nothing worked.

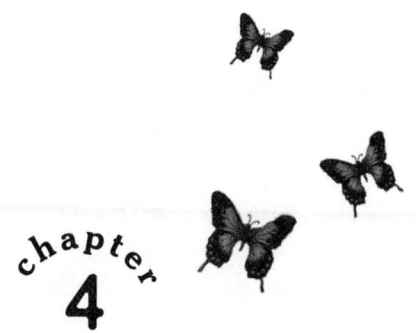

chapter 4

What is Alzheimer's Anyway?

This chapter is based on my twenty-year track record as a caregiver being with and around people said to be diagnosed with Alzheimer's. Mainstream medical science has different ways to talk about Alzheimer's and different facts to present. I'm not writing this as a doctor, since I'm not one, but as a practical caregiver and a longtime observer of the Alzheimer's scene.

So, what is Alzheimer's anyway? Alzheimer's is one form of dementia and there are many dementias and many causes of dementia, some of which we know and others we may not. Dementia is not a mental illness like schizophrenia or bipolar disorder, but an organic brain condition resulting from degenerative changes in the physical structure of the brain.

Although there are many kinds of dementia, you'll hear the name Alzheimer's more than any other right now. My own strong suspicion is that the word "Alzheimer's" is used far too often when it may not apply. After all, our Alzheimer's is *not* Dr. Alzheimer's Alzheimer's. The good doctor Alois Alzheimer (1864-1915) made a lifelong study of what was then called "pre-senile dementia" (what we would now call early-onset dementia) which affected people in their fifties and even their forties. His keynote case was a woman of fifty-one, brought to him suffering from severe memory issues, cognitive incapacity, and hallucinations.

Our modern Alzheimer's is said to affect about ten percent of people aged sixty-five and over, increasing to up to half of everyone aged eighty-five and over, even though the National Institute of Aging also says this is not a normal part of aging. Frankly, I find it hard to put those two concepts together – one in every two people has so-called Alzheimer's, and yet it is not a normal aging process.

If you are the child of a parent said to have Alzheimer's, you may become haunted by this possibility. Don't worry unnecessarily, but just understand how very loosely the term Alzheimer's is used. Right now there is no identifiable marker for Alzheimer's. Not even autopsy proves it infallibly, due to unaccounted-for discrepancies which appear in autopsied brains. An international conference of forensic experts in Berlin highlighted these as people diagnosed in life with dementia who did not have significant brain degeneration at autopsy, and people never diagnosed with dementia who did have significant degeneration of the physical brain.

There is not even a specific, proven gene connection. Some researchers are starting to talk about there being a whole variable group of Alzheimer's conditions. Other researchers explain that we are perhaps mistakenly grouping together a range of different conditions under the one heading of Alzheimer's. As a layperson, I'd go for that one. We know quite a bit about its processes but little about origins or treatment, all of which could change at any moment.

Alzheimer's tends to begin with minor memory issues or slight behavior oddities or changes that gradually accumulate in seriousness as not only memory but also cognitive and reasoning capacities become diminished. This is what we see from the outside. From within, it is likely that a person becomes aware much earlier on that something is wrong. In my experience of gathering evidence, people who are diagnosed in their sixties to seventies begin to be aware in their mid to late forties that there is something wrong. They may write about it in their own journals or letters, but they don't usually see doctors for it.

Alzheimer's is described as a terminal disease. Most people imagine a person ending up lying fetal, curled up in bed, neither speaking nor responding, and needing to be fed. And, moreover, if we listen enough to bad publicity, we are told that people with Alzheimer's lose all functions, become incontinent, and are pathetic, empty shells with nothing going on. Oh yes, *and* they get angry for no reason, wander, and have all kinds of weird, meaningless symptoms that cause trouble for others.

No wonder families despair once they hear the diagnosis of Alzheimer's. No wonder the adult children of parents with Alzheimer's feel threatened if they think of this as a possible future for themselves. However, many of those so-called facts are a kind of societal bigotry about dementia and are exaggerations and complete misunderstandings about people with dementia.

From my own observations and in my opinion, about ninety percent of those claimed to have Alzheimer's possibly do not. The medical profession's official claim is that Alzheimer's is accurately diagnosed in ninety percent of cases. Well, no. Dementia is, but Alzheimer's dementia is not. I can list ten common stress factors to be found in about ninety percent of people said to have Alzheimer's. Most are lifestyle stressors rather than organic or genetic causes.

I began to notice these stress factors myself as I gradually learned people's histories and made notes on them. As I travel giving workshops, I compare my checklist with other people's experiences in dementia and continue to find them universally applicable to the majority of people labeled as having Alzheimer's. That said, most dementias resemble each other and all dementias bring us similar problems and issues to deal with. Most of them right now are not treatable or curable, so maybe the name does not even matter.

However, to use a specific name like Alzheimer's, we need to be sure that this is what we're dealing with – and right now, we can't. Even the official diagnosis of Alzheimer's actually only means it is a dementia of the Alzheimer's type (DAT).

That diagnosis comes after extensive investigation has eliminated a number of other possible factors which could account for the appearance of dementia. You'll read every now and again that there is a definitive diagnostic test for Alzheimer's, but when you read the in-depth story under that newspaper headline, you'll find it's a diagnostic test that applies to most dementias. Every genetic clue that turns up also soon turns out to be irrelevant or only part of the story.

There are a number of familial early-onset dementias associated with specific chromosomes. Surely, instead of calling these Alzheimer's, should we not be calling them Chromosome 13 Dementia, Chromosome 14 Dementia, Chromosome 19 Dementia, and so on? A cynical researcher tells me that these are all lumped under the heading Alzheimer's because they were researched under Alzheimer's grants. If so, that does not help us get a true, clear picture of what Alzheimer's really is and how to diagnose it.

Perhaps in looking at so-called Alzheimer's, we are really looking at a storm of symptoms, behaviors, and physical changes that all have different origins and causes and are actually different conditions. Maybe we are in reality looking at an autoimmune condition, or series of conditions, which affects a person's immune system as it deteriorates sufficiently with age.

Some medical experts suggest that Alzheimer's itself is actually a whole group of dementias of various origins. Other than for fund-raising, it certainly doesn't matter much to caregivers. After all, what we have to deal with will be similar. Dementias have more in common than they have differences, and their differences give us little extra to work with as caregivers. They might be pointers for medical researchers but do not bring much light to caregiving.

Common Causes of Dementia

Since science isn't clarifying this much for us now, let me share my twenty years of observation with you. My guess is that most of those said to have Alzheimer's, a hauntingly scary disease of unknown origin, actually have dementia due to an accumulation of common causes. Again, from my own direct observations, plus input from many families as I've gone about the world giving workshops, I can list at least ten common issues that in my observation seem linked to the development of dementia. Of these, most people with intractable dementia usually notch up from five to ten of them. Here's the list:

1. Lack of Nurturing in Infancy and Early Childhood

The biggest single issue seems to be being born into a difficult family. This can be as varied as human situations are – being raised in a concentration camp, living in deprived family circumstances, possibly extreme poverty, mental health issues in a parent, alcoholism, abandonment, abuse, or any other factor which results in a person being deprived of emotional nourishment as an infant and young child.

This notably appears in at least ninety-five percent of everyone diagnosed with progressive dementia. It is very rare that someone who develops dementia after age sixty-five has *not* had this early childhood issue. Extreme poverty in itself is not a factor if nurturing was available. Adequate nurturing of an infant and toddler obviously safeguards that child in many ways from the effects of negative experiences.

This is not to say that everyone who has had such difficulties will inevitably develop incurable dementia. Not at all. It is the other way round – that we find that about ninety-five percent of everyone with progressive incurable dementia has had a challenging childhood experience.

What is the connection between late-in-life dementia and early lack of nurturing? Logically, from a physical point of view, we must assume that it is stress and the chemicals produced by it. Almost all major illness events are preceded by significant stress in most humans. Life observation and insurance companies tell us that.

We also know that stress attacks memory, either in a temporary way or, as in dementia, by doing permanent damage. Cortisol, the stress chemical, attacks choline, the memory chemical. We know this to be true in normal daily life for everyone. When you are under a lot of stress, no matter what your age, it's harder to remember things and to concentrate.

If you have had an entire lifetime of stress, it seems that being under attack so early in life may have created gateways into the immune system that later cause destruction in brain function. It is important to point out here that there may be nothing inevitable about this.

My first ten years of experience were almost exclusively with over-seventy-seven-year-olds up to ninety-seven-years-olds. That was a generation of people that did not get mental health therapy to deal with internal and emotional difficulties. Their stresses remained inside them, and I believe that this was the factor that set them up to be ideal candidates for dementia. By the time their dementia became outwardly apparent, the process of destruction was too well-established to be eradicable.

Many people don't realize this, but the beginning of what looks like later-life dementia is commonly experienced by people in their late forties. They may say nothing about it, but they are experiencing it in memory and thought issues.

I learned this from the first three people I cared for. One was a famous Jungian author and poet. She had a series of dreams in her mid-forties in which she was told that she had something wrong with her brain and that she was destined to join a special religious order, in the world but not of it. That's one of the best definitions of dementia I've ever heard.

The second person I knew had worked as a medical social worker and, in fact, became head of her department. She retired at sixty-five and was not diagnosed with Alzheimer's until her early eighties. However, when we cleared out her apartment after she moved into long-term care, I found a folder of yellowed newsprint articles dating from her late forties, all of them about memory problems. This was hidden in her underwear drawer.

The third person was seventy-four when she was diagnosed with Alzheimer's, and she had written in her diaries, which her family permitted me to read, references to "this terrible absent-mindedness of mine." She was forty-eight at the time she wrote those words. All of these experiences suggest to me that we should be checking in with people on memory issues much earlier than we do. Perhaps we could have more successful intervention. Medically speaking, this could be done especially with those known to have had early childhood deprivations.

2. Major Lifestyle Issues

There are no surprises here. These are the usual suspects in the development of poor health in later life. Poor diet, little exercise, addictions – these are all to be found as prevalent in those with dementia as those with other common health challenges.

3. Environmental Toxins

These include pollution, poisoning, and exposure to any other long-term degradation of the surrounding environment which affects health, or exposure to a short-term but major toxicity – anything from mercury poisoning to war toxins. Unfortunately, we may get the opportunity to see more of this with our returning Mid-East war veterans exposed to much toxicity.

4. Head Injuries

The Mayo Clinic reports that about one-third of everyone who has dementia has had a head injury earlier in life. It seems logical to assume that this also attacked the normal capacity of the brain to repair itself. Whether it is the head injury itself or the injury to the brain's capacity to stay healthy as age begins to weaken the immune system, we do not know.

Whether the exact nature of the head injury or the area injured is a factor, medical researchers have not yet fully established. As is so often the case, we need to see much more research undertaken so the answers to these questions can be found for future generations.

5. Medications

Everyone hates to admit this, but necessary, long-term use of powerful drugs can eventually bring about its own demand for payment. Something strong enough to radically control brain function may eventually bring about a functional link with dementia. For example, long-term users of prescribed tranquillizers and other mood-controlling medications may develop dementia, as well as those with anxiety issues who have become addicted to their medications. The medications for Parkinson's and seizure-control may also contribute to dementia.

Then there is the major issue of old age and prescription medications that can precipitate dementia. This can become even more contentious when the wrong kinds of medications are used to control people with dementia. Dr. Joe Graedon feels very strongly about this. He feels that the use of anti-psychotic medications on elders with dementia, simply for social control, is a public scandal. It is also illegal.

Long-term care staff use such medications because they say they work to control potentially difficult people, but then so would a two-by-four round the side of the head. Haldol is like a two-by-four when given to a confused elder, and I have witnessed at least one person who died from it.

Certain conditions require those drugs, and yet there are results that are more than just side effects. They eventually ruin lives. On the other hand, they give years of effective and rewarding life to people who need them. This does not include the average elder with dementia who has previously had no psychotic illnesses.

The average elder takes anywhere from six to fifteen different medications. None of them have been tested together. As far as I know, no official scientific body is correlating the cumulative effects of these combinations. Therefore, it is up to the responsible caregiver – YOU – to note what happens with medications and changes of medication. Keep a medication journal in which you note new adverse developments, talk to a pharmacist, and then take the information to your elder's doctor.

Be as firm as you need to be to get that doctor's attention. If necessary, do what we had to do when running our care home – dispense with a doctor who did not listen or who even denied the manufacturer's actual listed side effects. You pay doctors plenty – make sure you get consumer satisfaction. Don't feel shy about it. Remember – what you don't speak up about could kill an elder you care about.

6. Surgery and General Anesthesia

Most people know by now that it is a risky business to undergo general anesthesia, especially if you are aged sixty and over. One statistic often quoted is that about thirty-three percent of people who undergo open-heart surgery or similarly lengthy operations experience a permanent drop in cognitive and memory function. There have been hundreds of medical studies conducted by research doctors which support this statistic. Again, of course, people need to weigh the gain against the risk and make a fully informed decision. After all, as one surgeon told me, "There's nothing like being dead to give you a really bad memory!"

Amongst those I've known with dementia, a significant number of them had undergone at least two operations involving the use of general anesthesia when over the age of sixty-five. In some cases, they might have been able to avoid this had they been fully informed or had they questioned their surgeons about the necessity for intervention.

Remember, it is in the nature of a surgeon to cut. That is what a surgeon does. Therefore, you must become informed about the need for and possible results of a surgery. Read everything you can on the Internet or get someone to get that information for you. Get a second opinion and even a third. It is absolutely necessary for you to understand a medical condition and its treatments and then make your own decision about it. Doctors are experts on conditions, yes, but you and you alone are the expert on who will make choices for the person you care for.

These days, many surgeons tend to offer other alternatives for elders undergoing necessary procedures. For example, many hip replacement procedures are now done under sedation of a different kind, for this very reason. You should always ask if there is a comfortable alternative to general anesthesia. Apparently some surgeons are still in denial about this, but any online search on general anesthesia and cognitive impairment will bring up hundreds of reports. Print them out and wave them under your surgeon's nose.

7. Cumulative Trauma in Old Age

Insurance actuary tables show that stressful events are often the forerunner of severe illnesses or accidents, and we see this constantly born out in the lives of elders. Elder mental-health care has been pretty much ignored as a factor in the development of dementia, but it is often the case that elders experience a series of traumatic events in fairly short succession.

Maybe they have been relocated when they did not want to be, have experienced the death of a spouse or other family member, were involved in a car accident, or were the victim of a crime. Given the general lack of peer-group support systems, an older person can be left feeling seriously traumatized with no support to promote emotional recovery.

It would be comparatively easy and inexpensive for any community to start support groups for elders recovering from traumatic events, and it is possible that such groups would be able to prevent some people from failing into a dementia state. There are grief support groups, but not trauma or distress groups.

8. Undiagnosed, Lifelong Mental Illness

Members of this group may not be as numerous as those in the other categories, yet I have found this to be a small but significant group that is very seldom talked about.

In my first dementia-care home-management job, two out of five residents were actually not affected much by dementia but were notably mentally ill. While trying not to actually diagnose them myself, I noticed they both expressed peculiar paranoid fantasies and either a high fear or anger response to much of life. One heard voices; the other had anger attacks and was violent.

They were both experienced by their families as difficult, hard-to-handle women and were somewhat estranged from their own children. In both cases, the daughters had left the administration of their mothers' affairs to the grown grandchildren. I was very struck by the fact that two out of five residents were so affected and thereafter looked out for other examples of this.

Since then, I can affirm that this is a significant though small group that can be found in every so-called Alzheimer's or dementia residence. Apparently, families are reluctant to push for mental health intervention for parents who have been functional but difficult throughout their lives.

Sometimes the family has probably not clearly identified that their elder is mentally ill, and, in other cases, perhaps the shame of such identification prevents the elder from getting appropriate help. Such people tend to be easily classified as having Alzheimer's when bizarre behaviors in old age get them sent to long-term care without much investigation.

Every Alzheimer's unit usually has a group of residents who are mentally ill much more than demented, and it makes me wonder what the true figures actually are. My guess is that about two out of ten of all people said to have Alzheimer's are more likely to be suffering from a longtime mental illness and not the organic disease of dementia.

9. Dietary Dementia

This can be the result of lifelong poor dietary habits, the development of such habits in old age, or changes in the body chemistry and functional abilities as a result of failing health in old age. For example, it is very common for people to be vitamin deficient, and there are dementias associated specifically with these deficiencies. Sometimes paying attention to this can reduce or even completely dissipate the effects of such deficiency.

Another issue very seldom spoken of is the lack of digestive enzymes in elders which leads to nutritional deficiency even when they may actually be eating good food often enough. Without sufficient digestive enzymes, for example, the complex sugars that the brain requires for adequate functioning cannot reach the brain and it will not be able to function well.

In our care home, we had the experience of giving digestive enzymes to one resident and seeing a huge improvement in her wakefulness, cognition, and intellectual engagement with life. It did not improve her memory but it improved brain function overall.

10. Undiagnosed Adult-Onset Hydrocephalus

Hydrocephalus in older adults is a neurological disorder in which an excess of cerebrospinal fluid accumulates in the brain, creating dangerous pressure – "water on the brain" as people popularly and not quite accurately used to call it. It is caused by a gradual shrinkage of the pathways which formerly drained the fluid away safely. This can be the result of strokes, the actual shrinkage of the entire brain, or other factors of old age.

The symptoms of such a condition may include vomiting, nausea, severe headaches, sleeping too much, seizures, visual disturbances, memory loss, gait disorder, urinary incontinence, and a general slowing of activity, as well as apparent dementia.

Opinion is gathering to suggest that many cases of so-called Alzheimer's may actually be adult-onset hydrocephalus, which occurs in adults over sixty. Medical investigation can establish whether that is so, using any or all of the following – ultrasound, CAT scan, MRI, lumbar puncture or tap, and intra-cranial pressure monitoring. The usual treatment seems to be inserting an artificial pressure shunt, which is usually rated by surgeons as minimally invasive and seems to have a lot of success at low risk.

The after-effects of the procedure can be a considerable reduction in what were formerly assumed to be Alzheimer's symptoms. It does not remove all symptoms of dementia, but it seems to allow a much more competent lifestyle to reassert itself in this person.

I urge everyone to make sure any elder with apparent dementia have an Alzheimer's work-up with the brain pressure test as well. I personally know two people who benefited from this and I now hear about others all the time. It is not a significantly difficult ordeal, considering the enormous potential benefits. The results can bring about a much higher quality of life for an elder. If your neurologist or Alzheimer's diagnostic center does not suggest this, ask. If they don't provide it, find someone who does and get a really informed expert opinion on it.

11. Dementia of the Dying Process

This is much ignored by the medical profession and unknown to family members. The main reason why so much dementia – allegedly fifty percent of all elders – is seen in the eighty-five-and-older set is that they are walking the pathway to death. After all, let's be real here, most people are dead by eighty-four.

It is really quite rare for an older person to fall to the ground dead of a heart attack. Mostly, the path of dying is gradual, involving a slow attrition of health due to whatever systems are failing the most, and then perhaps a period of time spent in bed doing the actual dying. Most elders die very peacefully, these days often helped and supported by the wonderful Hospice workers who also support, guide, and help family members through the unfamiliar process.

In the months or even years of walking towards death, the majority of elders will experience a gradual reduction of former function. Maybe they don't walk so well or eat so heartily, and they often experience the kind of brain function changes that we recognize as dementia. This is not, however, Alzheimer's. It is a dementia of the dying process that comes about because all functions of this old body are now beginning to decline. It is very normal for most people.

We can choose to see this as sad or pitiable, but there are other ways we can choose to see the dementia of the dying process. I see it as a way that this person can give less time to the practicalities of living and more time to the dreams, memories, and life story of this lifetime. Brain studies of people with dementia show they have a very active dream life. It is not surprising to me that this is when the dead relatives start to visit – Uncle Harry, Mom, a deceased husband. These are not hallucinations or a sign of craziness. These experiences occur within every culture in the whole of humankind, which suggests to me these are the natural processes of a person moving towards death.

I'm not a theologian nor a psychologist, so I can't tell you how this person truly experiences these events. Are they really the return of the spirits of dear ones who have died before, gathering to comfort this family member or waiting to take them safely to the life of the spirit? Beats me, folks. Maybe.

Or maybe this is intense memory recall at work, flashbacks so real to this person that they feel the presence and hear the voice of those they loved and lost from their life. Maybe this is how the human being is equipped to take the death journey, so that this person can comfort him- or herself with waking dreams. Maybe the closing down of the brain changes brain chemistry so much that they experience an entirely different way of communicating with the whole of creation, memory, and their own consciousness.

Whatever it is, it's normal. Most old and dying people have experiences of this kind. It brings comfort and ease to a difficult process, so heck – I say, enjoy it all. Don't call in the psychiatrist. Don't drug the person out of the experiences. Sit and hold their hand, talk kindly, and be there, as human beings have sat beside each other for the many, many centuries of our existence.

What if It's Really Alzheimer's?

The main thing to draw from all these experiences, and the many things that will happen in your caregiving, is to trust your own knowing. Try not to become distressed about dementia. Just take it day by day. Cut out those articles on new developments, but don't believe everything you read. Keep hoping, though, because this is the most-researched illness on the planet. Hope keeps you realizing that everything can heal, and really being awake to your own process and experiences as a caregiver will gradually teach you that much can be healed that cannot necessarily be cured.

That is the essential teaching within any illness, any disease process, or any injury to health. There is a road to knowledge that is linked to our spiritual growth and healing when we stop fighting the process and become willing to take it day by day and learn from what we see.

There is one more thing you should know about dementia. Everyone does dementia in his or her own way. While the central issues probably affect everyone – memory problems, for example – the ways they develop, the losses that materialize, the symptoms that appear are very variable indeed. One person might lose the power of speech very early in their dementia. Someone else might early on forget how to read and write.

Another person might simply begin showing memory problems and a little cognitive impairment.

Dementia is not really an exact process; it is more an entire syndrome, which usually starts slowly and almost imperceptibly. Over the months and years that follow, a cascade of other impairments occurs, again different for different people. It is not true that the inevitable end of Alzheimer's is a person lying fetal and unable to speak in a bed, needing hand feeding. Oddly enough, in those people it might happen fairly early on and they might live for six or seven years in that state. It is an unusual variation affecting about three percent of everyone diagnosed or said to have Alzheimer's, so this does not in fact represent a true picture of general dementia. Most who have Alzheimer's die of the normal health conditions of old age – heart disease or cancer or stroke.

Of course, what a list of symptoms can never do is to show how the person is doing within that framework of symptoms. Is this person happy, frightened, developing spiritually? None of that is included in a typical medical analysis. Later we'll explore further the question of how people with dementia may grow even within the framework of an illness that diminishes their normal life.

Just know for the moment that happiness, love, and laughter can occur regularly in the daily life of a person with dementia and that part of your job as a caregiver is to enhance these opportunities and enjoy them yourself.

A LIFE IN ALZHEIMER'S LAND

To make a successful working relationship with Hannah required the ability to be in the present moment and to concentrate on heart connection. It was a state of being with her that was required, not a state of doing to her. There was something clearly meditative about the way I had to be with Hannah if our relationship was to work.

Once I realized that, I found it very peaceful to be there.

We had our difficulties, of course. One was the teeth. Hannah had false teeth which had to be soaked overnight. The first time I helped her go to bed, I said, "Okay, Hannah, time to take out your teeth."

"My teeth?" she said wonderingly. "I cannot. They are my own teeth."

"Yes, I know they are – but they come out."

"No, they do not. They are mine."

"They are not your teeth. You always take them out and put them in the glass there." I pointed.

"But that is impossible."

"It's not impossible. Your teeth don't grow there. They're false teeth." I was starting to sweat now.

"Ach! You're crazy!" she said. Eventually, she took them out, but it was the first of many such occasions.

chapter 5

Making Sense of Dementia

There really is sense in dementia. You really can make a survival plan for your energy, your commonsense, your sense of humor, and your ability to hope. And you'll pick up lots of caregiving shortcuts that will keep your elder safe and you sane.

How dementia affects a person is usually the most difficult aspect of this illness for caregivers because we usually take a while to understand how it operates. So I'm going to save you some bemusement time. The usual problems of dementia are:

- Memory glitches

- Loss of ability to think rationally

- The way physical and emotional feelings are interpreted by the body, heart, and spirit of a person with dementia

These problems can manifest in many ways and we can never guess in advance exactly how those complications will surface. One of the things I love about people with Alzheimer's is that they will make up life as they go along. This means they are seldom boring, but it is exactly what makes so many problems for us caregivers.

If we allow it, we can experience this as one of the greatest frustrations of caregiving. Smart caregivers, however, make a healthy decision not to feel crazy just because their elder seems to be trying to make them so. In fact, many of the apparent oddities of dementia make a certain sense once you can guess at what is going on.

"My mother can remember all kinds of things about her childhood. Yet, if I ask her about her day, she doesn't seem to remember anything."

This is a typical complaint caregivers bring to workshops and there are two aspects to it. One is that memory does have its own strange manifestations in dementia. The second is that the caregiver keeps suspecting that the person with dementia might actually be doing this stuff deliberately. To stay sane, *never assume an elder with dementia is trying to drive you crazy.*

First, a person with dementia can't plan this because memory issues don't allow the logical making and carrying through of plans. Second, get a grip on your own emotions. Someone has to stay sensible, rational, and calm in a dementia situation – and that someone has to be you.

So let's make sane guesses about what goes on in memory issues for an elder with dementia. Remember that science is only beginning to unravel the mysteries of memory. Much remains unknown and new discoveries are being made all the time, so our caregiver guesses are as good as anything else. Current scientific opinion seems to be that memory is stored in different parts of the brain. Short-term memory is the most afflicted form of memory in those with dementia and is thought to be stored in the hippocampus, an area usually heavily affected by plaques and tangles.

Having dementia means that the normal routines of the brain can no longer operate in the same way they used to, due to the physical degeneration of the brain system. Short-term memory fails greatly and, with that, so do the usual habits of life. When we cannot rely on short-term memory, our sense of our own story begins to fragment. When that happens, we also begin to fragment. How we experience ourselves is what makes us who we are, and remembering who we are is an important part of that.

According to the latest studies of brain operation, it takes about two hours for an experience to go from the short-term sector of memory to being lodged permanently in the long-term sector, which is exactly why people with dementia have such trouble telling you about their day. They cannot hold a short-term memory item long enough for that to happen. That means when you ask them in the evening what they did that day, the information has vanished from short-term memory and has never been stored in long-term memory.

For most human beings, losing their story is an emotional wound. Our story sets us in the center of our life. It gives us relevance, power, and a good sense of self. If you doubt that, think of all those movies where the hero wakes up in a hotel room and has amnesia. The rest of the movie is a frantic search for his identity. Finding his identity will reveal to him who he is and how he lives. And we need this information for our emotional and mental health.

When that is eroded by dementia, it is very distressing for most people. It makes them frightened, lonely, and bewildered. Very few people are centered well enough in their deep, unchanging spiritual self to not worry. Those who lose memory reliability deal with it in a number of ways. They may supply information from their overall intuitive sense/feeling of what daily life is like. So, your mother – who's been at home all day – may say, "I went shopping and had lunch with my friend Amy; then we saw a movie." All fictional.

She says this because she cannot recall what she did, but she has a sense of what life might have been on an average day. Does she know she's lying, or "confabulating" as psychiatrists like to call it? Hard to say, but probably not. She's just giving a reasonable account of life according to how she probably always lived it.

You might do the same if someone asked you if you had breakfast yesterday. You would answer based on what you know to be your usual routine and maybe only later recall that you had to leave early and couldn't make time for breakfast. Did you lie? Not really. Well, that's also what happens for the person working inside the loss of short-term memory.

Short-term memory damage means losing recent events, even as little as five minutes ago, but there are a lot of variables. Some short-term memory events might be remembered for hours, even days. Always assume that any memory issue is due to the dementia. Don't choose to get into blame – "she could have remembered that if she wanted to" – since you'll never know the truth. No point in tormenting yourself.

Long-term memories go back as far in life as people can remember clearly – usually somewhere between two and four years old – and in the person with Alzheimer's these memories tend to be as accurate or inaccurate as the memories of anyone without Alzheimer's. In other words, they may stay intact or they may get fuzzy, having nothing to do particularly with dementia, but just with the normal human memory variants.

To me, one of the most interesting aspects of Alzheimer's is that people with dementia almost always go and live, as it were, in other time zones. For example, Austin, Texas, 1929. Your mom expects her parents to be home for dinner and she thinks she has homework from school to do. She knows who's alive in 1929 and can name them all. *You* are assigned the name of the relative you most resemble, or interestingly, maybe the role name "Mom." These voyages down the river of time are obviously, at one level, due to short-term memory impairment. Your mom does not remember what year this is.

However, it is also apparent to me that people go to these other time zones in order to undertake some uncompleted task around life issues. In that time zone, there is still meaningful work to be done, psychological processes to be completed, and something to be experienced that this person has not yet finished in their heart and spirit. This great purposeful journeying seems to have been largely ignored by the dementia community – whether the medical side or the caregiver side – but it is part of what I would call the sacred work of aging. This is what people without dementia do in old age as well. Old men and women are greatly absorbed in their life journey, especially with what happened in their early life. We seem to have ignored the *why* of all this.

It is not the aimless musing of people locked into the past. For all human beings, the most powerful and important life experiences tend to happen in the first twenty years of life. True, other big experiences will be added – war, childbirth, challenges of various natures. But it is our formative years, containing our making, our wounding, and our awakenings, that essentially form who we are. To complete our soul journey, we have to deeply examine them and how we have learned, grown, changed, or remained wounded or childlike. We have to know at the deepest level how we became who we became and what life path resulted from that. We have to wake up.

For me, one of the most profound gifts of dementia is that it allows an elder to revisit these issues with a deep involvement in them. Often, people with dementia have lived notably stressful and demanding lives, with no time for this deep journeying. What the world sees as their illness can also be, in its odd way, a blessing. They have time at last. People with poor short-term memory are in every way able to do that sacred work. They are working at finding peace and resolution in their life journey. I explore this more fully in Chapter Nine.

So I suggest you support this great work. Instead of worrying that your mother doesn't know her mother is dead, and calls you by her brother's name, just be willing to sit with her in that time. When you see an opportunity, just enter it. "So what's your mom like?" you could ask. Or, "What do you think is for dinner?"

These openings will encourage your elder to explore more of that time, to talk about people who probably haven't been talked about for a long time. Maybe, if you're very blessed, you'll begin to find out why your mother has to return there. What work remains to be done? She might reveal old wounds or loss or sorrow and, if this happens, you are truly blessed because you will be her true companion on the dementia journey. The loneliness of dementia is so profound because no one values the memories or the attempts to make things right within their own hearts.

If you can support this process, *you* are a great soul. You will always cherish and honor anything revealed to you in this way. There are some caregiver dilemmas around these issues, though. People wonder if they should remind their mother that her mother is long dead. Is it wrong not to do this? Will it confuse your mother's ability to know what is what, if you don't remind her? Will you be making her illness worse if you don't try to keep her tied to present day reality?

These are good questions. Answer number one: there is hardly anything you can do which will make dementia better or worse. You can make the person you look after feel better or worse, but we don't really have much control over the course of their illness. Answer number two: you probably won't be able to persuade a person living in a different time zone in their hearts that today is a different time and place anyway.

They are more likely to think that *you* are the crazy one. If you tell them their mother is dead, they are more likely to scream, "What! What happened to her? I just saw her half an hour ago! Oh my God!" and then you'll really feel bad because your good intentions made your mother cry.

Understand that as long as your elder deeply feels that this is 1929, it will be until he or she is ready to let go of it. This tends to be fairly short-term – maybe an hour or so, more or less. You'll notice when your mother has come back to this time zone. Just do what you do, carry on as normal, because what you're seeing *is* normal for short-term memory loss. There's nothing to worry about. Be kind and break out those cookies after a while.

Three-Way Triage

Now let's consider an issue usually seen as major by caregivers and figure out a solution. Since it is the lack of apparent order that drives most caregivers crazy, it can be very useful to bring your own order to problems you encounter.

When faced with a problem, try to classify the importance and urgency of action necessary, just the way medical personnel do at the scene of an accident. They have to triage it and make decisions about the nature of the help to be given. You could do the same for problem behaviors. Think about triaging in one of three ways.

1. Urgent! *Must* take action because of possible danger resulting from a behavior. An example of this would be your father leaving the house in the middle of the night to walk down the nearby freeway, just because he feels the urge to walk and he's always more active at night. You would call 911 instantly. You would go in pursuit, because he could be hit by a car and killed or could wander away, never to be seen alive again.

Once you get him back safely, you have subsidiary actions to take. Secure the house so he can no longer leave without your knowledge. Install an alarm system and security locks, consider having someone come in for night duty, and make a new plan to exhaust your dad in the daytime so he might sleep at night. Consider asking his doctor if sleep medication is appropriate – not my favorite thing but sometimes the only safe choice.

2. Not urgent, but still necessary to take some action. For example, every afternoon around 4.30 p.m. your mom gets restless and emotional, sometimes anxious, sometime angry. This is her sun-downing pattern (described in Chapter Six) and you have choices about what to do. You could, in the short-term, divert her by taking her out for a drive in the car, for example. You could ignore her, knowing that this agitation will pass, and be secure in knowing that you don't have to be agitated as well. Or you could make a plan to change things in the future by learning what sun-downing is, how to work with it, and how to bring about lasting changes.

3. No action necessary. Your aunt keeps going through the drawers one by one, sometimes taking things out, sometimes not. It annoys you. Probably your aunt is either under-amused or is handling her anxieties by doing this. After you've made sure there is nothing essential in those drawers that she could remove, let her do what she does. Choose not to be annoyed by her fidgeting. You might devise more entertainment for her, or you might accept that this is actually her hobby now and let it go.

Triaging helps you bring order to situations. There is really only one burden related to a difficult behavior and that is making a decision about it. However, if you get tired or overwhelmed, it is easy to add a second unnecessary burden and this is the one that kills caregivers. It is your attitude burden – anger, despair, and irritation. Understandable, but you do have the power to choose to set them aside. Give yourself a break.

You do not have to bite that hook, as the fine Buddhist nun Pema Chodron says in her teachings. As a caregiver, it is important to save your energy for when it's needed. Do not get caught up in the situation as if your feelings were the reality of what is going on. They come, they go, they are merely reactions. You can learn to master them, meditatively.

Three-Point-Plan

Before we look at the classic so-called difficult behaviors of Alzheimer's, let me introduce you to the Three-Point-Plan (I like to call this the Fabulous Frena Three-Point-Plan – but then I would, wouldn't I?), a formula whereby you will be able to decode most behaviors and understand how you can approach the necessary problem-solving. The plan is just three questions to ask yourself. Do this when you are facing a behavior that causes problems for the well-being, safety, or welfare of someone you're caring for. Remember that triaging has shown us that a problem that merely bothers you doesn't need to be dealt with. You just need an attitude adjustment. (See Chapter Seven for self-care ideas.)

Here are the three questions to ask yourself when considering a problem behavior:

1. What is the feeling underlying this behavior?

2. What is the unmet need underlying this feeling?

3. How can we meet this need?

Let's take a hard-to-solve problem as an example. Your mother comes up to you and says, "Where's my mother?" Apply the questions.

From your answers, you might reasonably guess that (1) your mother *feels* as if she is indeed a motherless child. (2) She *needs* mother-like care in this moment. (3) *You can do that*, even if you're a guy.

So you answer her question with a useful and yet truthful evasion. "Gee, I don't know where your mother is right now." What? You were about to tell this needing-to-be-mothered person that her mother is dead? I don't think so. Then you put your arm around her, lead her somewhere comfortable, and sit together with cookies and a drink. What often seem to be great unsolvable problems most often come down to reassuringly kind actions. The language of our physical actions can be gift enough.

A LIFE IN ALZHEIMER'S LAND

I was fascinated by Hannah's dilemma. She had no reliable access to her own memories. It meant not only that her own life history was fractured, but that she had lost the means to organize her own present. Knowing to bathe, to dress, how to cook, simply knowing what comes next or what happened yesterday – it was all gone.

I wondered sometimes if it was like wandering in a huge empty warehouse, opening doors and finding deserted rooms, or perhaps it was like opening your safe deposit box to find everything taken. We are so used to thinking it is our mind which guards all our treasures. However, I was also finding the opposite in living with Hannah – that we have valuables in our hearts and senses, too. We are still a person, just a very different person.

She had a full heart and she had a gift that her illness could give us. She was completely accepting of us, warm, easily amused, undemanding. Her love was just a flow, not a condition of exchange or an artificial sweetener. She was who she was, we were who we were; that was enough.

Daily Dementia, or Why is S/he Doing That?

Caregivers worry more about behaviors than people with dementia do, most of the time. Unless actual risk is involved, we caregivers could decide to just let most of these issues go. We could, but we don't. We could say, like a mantra, "It's her illness, it's his Alzheimer's," but we don't.

So, because we don't, I'm going to share the observations I have on the most common behavioral issues that bother caregivers. Some include a list of possible solutions; others are simply reminders to you that all is not well; and others – well, they really don't matter. Little children will sometimes sing endlessly in an irritating way and it doesn't matter. What are you going to do – beat them, send them for singing lessons? Ideally, neither. You're going to let them do what they're doing.

This is often true of the typical dementia behaviors. Like children, people with dementia are seeking consolation, amusement, healing, or are working out some inner issue through what they express. There is an integrity of action which results in behaviors which this person uses to find healing. Since they have dementia, it can be a very roundabout journey.

Here are some of the most annoying common behaviors caregivers deal with.

Agitation

Life is hard to understand when you have dementia because it takes time to mentally process what is happening. Therefore, a person may become agitated because of fear, a sudden event (like being soaked by a sprinkler hose), adverse weather conditions like wind (to which elders with dementia are very sensitive), trying to hurry the person, sun-downing, or because of some inner thought you can't even guess at.

Someone has to stand calm against agitation, and that would be you. Agitated feelings are contagious; so when the person you care for is agitated, don't get caught up in it. Breathe deeply, stay calm, and say something soothing like, "Let's go and sit down out of the rain."

If agitation actually becomes a tantrum, stand further back to give this person space and wait it out. If people look at you, say, "My mother has Alzheimer's and she gets upset sometimes." They will look sympathetic and vanish at speed. Remember, you don't actually have to do anything about agitation. It's just a feeling and it doesn't do any harm. Keep breathing calmly and deeply. As soon as the right moment comes, say cheerfully, "Okay then, let's go home now, shall we?"

It is rare for a person with dementia to strike out, run away, or be physically aggressive while upset. You just have to give them space, ignore the bystanders, and get the heck out of Dodge as soon as you can. Most agitation passes quickly. Remember, you usually cannot re-train a person with dementia. Learn what the triggers are and avoid them as far as possible.

Agitation on a regular basis at a regular time is probably sun-downing, a period of agitation most common towards the end of the day. See *sun-downing* below.

Anger

People talk about the anger of people with dementia as though it were a mysterious, unaccountable emotion under the circumstances. Yet, back in the 1950s, Doctor Elisabeth Kübler-Ross was already detailing the lives and reactions of people with terminal illnesses. Among their usual reactions was – yes – *anger*. Yet most professionals still don't seem to get the connection.

I suspect this is because we think people with dementia can't remember to be angry. But those patients of Kübler -Ross were not angry through memory, reason, or logic. Their anger was an organic response to the fear and feeling of how it is to be dying. So, too, are people with Alzheimer's. They are besieged by something that will not let them go, which steals their normal life away and leaves them bereft. Who wouldn't be angry? It is a totally normal response to the onset of incurable illness.

This kind of anger tends to appear most severely in the early stages of dementia when the person is aware that there is trouble within and feels upset, fearful, and agitated. If this person is also being secretive, then it may appear as sudden unexpected outbursts of rage.

If an older person you know is having apparent personality changes of this kind, it is time to get them to a doctor. Once you know this is part of dementia, choose to understand angry or mean outbursts as fearfulness.

The other anger we hear of is the anger of so-called combativeness. A husband is upset. A good caring wife moves in to soothe him and BAM! If a man with dementia is angry, it is wiser to step back out of fist range and literally give him space to have his feelings and collect himself again. Don't try to soothe, but instead validate.

"Of course you're upset..." is a good start, and don't stand too close. That is not what a besieged person wants. People with dementia get angry because something happens that frightens them. Typically a man may strike out with his fist; a woman may cry.

Combativeness is the result of overwhelming feelings of fear. My experience of this kind of rage at home is that it is often associated with family secrecy. No one wants to talk about dementia, yet this person always knows that something is wrong. Fear diminishes when it can be talked about.

If someone doesn't want to admit having dementia, let it be. That denial is fear. The safer a person feels, the more likely that reluctance will go away. Meanwhile, you can't win an argument about it, so let it go.

In a care facility, violence typically happens in the bathroom or during a shower, both occasions when a guy expects to be alone and not have bossy strangers getting into the act. My experience is that care staff always know what triggers the anger, yet they still do it. Unfortunately, it is the resident who gets blamed and often punitively medicated, even though this is supposed to be illegal now. Since bathroom and shower use has long been private in this resident's life, a staff member needs to be polite, move slow, and ask permission – *yes*, every time. Why? Because having dementia often means starting life anew every day.

Every care action taken by staff needs to enhance this person's fragile sense of security, not demolish it. Softness, politeness, and slowness all reassure the frightened resident. Remember the Biblical injunction – "A soft answer turneth away wrath." (Proverbs 15:1)

If someone who was always calm and agreeable starts throwing objects at the wall one day, don't call a psychiatrist. Instead call the doctor, because it may well mean there is another physical or medical condition developing. Some care facilities, unfortunately, do not always understand this. They might say your elder has become violent overnight. Not true. There may be something physically wrong and this person needs to see a doctor immediately, and you need a better care place for your elder.

Bathing

Many families become concerned that an elder with Alzheimer's is no longer taking showers and indeed seems to be resisting them altogether. It is certainly true that many elders with dementia develop what looks like a fear of showers and we can only guess why. Maybe the feeling of water striking the head is unwelcome, painful even. Maybe they forget how to take a shower and it is all too daunting.

Don't worry, your elder will not die of grubbiness and, in fact, the skin of older people does not do too well with frequent showering. So the number of showers can certainly be reduced as long as daily sponge bathing happens.

Another way to handle this is to use a hand-held shower and help the person bathe by starting at the feet and working your way up. Avoid watering the top of the head altogether during most shower-times. Often it's better to have a hairdresser wash this person's hair since that is usually experienced as a familiar, non-threatening routine, especially for women. It evokes life as it used to be.

Consider getting someone to come in and bathe your elder using the hand-held shower. Home health aides are very good at this and it is no hassle for them. It can be a good investment of your resources and may even be a free service if you qualify.

Unless someone has a serious hygiene problem because of being unable to complete cleaning up after using the toilet, a twice-weekly shower can be sufficient. For the rest of the week, a fresh washcloth and verbal instruction can do the job.

Many people who originally preferred actual baths may begin taking showers instead. Access to a shower is easier and they can sit on a shower chair whilst doing the job. No one whose balance is uncertain should continue to use a bathtub. Even with supplemental handrails, the risk of falling is too great. Once dementia becomes an issue, you can never be sure that a person is able to manage safe use of a bathtub.

Changes in a person's visual-spatial abilities make use of tubs and even accurate placement on the toilet hazardous. No one knows whether this is an actual change in the brain's capacity to estimate how to place the body, or whether it is the person being less able to compute it. Whichever it is, a caregiver will need to carefully monitor how this person sits on the shower chair and on the toilet seat. Physical guidance works best for this. Most caregivers give a gentle maneuver in the right direction at the right moment to get someone seated safely.

Verbal cues don't seem that effective. "Careful! Watch out!" seems useless, probably because this person doesn't think they're doing anything dangerous.

Choices

You want to empower but not confuse people who have dementia. When a decision is to be made, give two choices but not more, as in "Would you like this red sweater or this blue one?" while waving each sweater at the appropriate verbal cue. Having the appearance of choice is pleasing to them as they often feel helpless and controlled by others.

People with dementia get tired of never being able to do what they want, so try to find as many ways to empower them as possible, within the limits of their capacity to manage. When asking what they would choose, show the choices. Many people have forgotten what nouns mean. Make your suggestions in question form, such as, "Would you like to go for a ride in the car?"

On the other hand, do *not* give choices where you really do not want the answer "No!" Don't ask your father if he would like to get ready to go the doctor's office if you don't want a refusal. Opinions vary on how to deal with these issues, but I'm all for not facing issues before we face them.

Therefore, if I had to get my mother to the doctor's office for an appointment, I'd get her up and organized in easy time and then I'd get her into the car, all without even mentioning doctor or appointment. I would not actually lie, because I don't believe in that, but I would omit full information. "Let's go for a ride!" I'd say cheerfully.

Then I would drive to the doctor's office and we'd get out and then we'd walk into the office – surprise! Same for any other possibly unwelcome journey. Going to day-care, for example. I would never pre-announce this if I thought it would be unpopular.

You might like the idea of full disclosure right now as you read this, but I guarantee you won't always feel that way. Yes, it is manipulation, but that is one of our useful management tools in dementia care. My motto is, "Never lie, but do not always tell the whole truth during the average dementia day."

Communication

Brain changes may demand that you change the way you communicate with your elder. All kinds of difficulties can occur. It is not unusual for people to begin to forget the connection between a noun and the object it names. I first experienced this with Hannah.

"Could I have that knife, please, Hannah?" I asked one day, pointing vaguely towards her side of the table. She passed, in turn, a sugar bowl, a saltcellar, and an envelope before I realized she had no idea what the word "knife" meant. I pointed straight to the knife after that.

One man at day-care told me angrily about his wife. "I must have told her about six times to switch off the light!" he snorted. And he looked shocked when I suggested she might no longer know what the word "light" referred to. This loss of nouns is not uncommon and ultimately often extends also to proper nouns, that is, people's names.

Communication needs to be simpler with dementia – one idea at a time and spoken in a clear, unhurried way, preferably when you are seated at the same level as the person you are talking to. Looming over them or talking loudly can be interpreted as hostile or threatening. If people become afraid, they also become fear-deaf and don't hear or respond to what you say.

Give directions one step at a time, and wait for their response before you go on to the next step. Point to the objects you are referring to. Take time. Be calm. Don't patronize. A person with dementia can smell patronage at ten thousand yards.

Verbal cueing for getting dressed might sound like this. "So, here's your clothes. All clean and fresh. Why don't you put this shirt on first? That's great. Here, let me help you with the sleeves. Good. How about the pants? Tell you what. You sit so I can help you get them on your legs. Here we go, one foot, now the other foot, that's great. Why don't you stand up, then you can pull them up. Yes, that's really good. You need to zip them up – don't want to get those ladies out there too excited."

I often joke a lot when I'm working with someone. It has less edge than giving people orders. You need to take your time doing all this without impatience, which is why I'll patter on with remarks and jokes as I verbally cue every step of dressing. If someone can dress himself or herself, then I will always let them do it, even if it takes a while. If I were an impatient home caregiver, and I have been one, I might take a book or newspaper in with me since I would have something else to do while going through the process.

"Why don't you sit down again? That's good. Now, here's your socks. Here's the first one. Oh, that's looks good on your hand but actually it's better for keeping your foot warm. Yes, that foot. Now, how about the other foot? Here we go," and so on in amiable soothing babble.

Our aim is to help and guide, not humiliate. After all, if people could dress themselves, obviously they would.

Dehydration

Most elders drink less water than they should, which is why so many have constipation. It is water alone that can fix that problem.

Drinking enough fluids is vitally important because the level of dementia can be affected by dehydration. An elder with dementia will become more confused and less responsive when dehydrated. At least four eight-ounce measures of water a day are needed, more if possible.

Put the water into small glasses, which seem less intimidating to elders with dementia, and keep renewing them. Remind the person to take a little drink, often. Make a game of this. If necessary, splash just enough juice into it to make it look and taste better. If there is afternoon confusion, be sure to increase fluid intake because this can make a significant improvement.

Some elders are reluctant to drink much water either because they never did or because they feel it will make them go to the bathroom more – which is true. Just encourage them with lots of good humor. Try bribery, persuasion, and reward, and remind them the doctor wanted them to drink plenty.

Driving

In my opinion, driving is never to be done by someone with dementia. Recent studies have shown that of every ten people with dementia still driving, five have had really serious accidents in which they killed or badly injured someone, and three more have had multiple fender-benders and more. Families are very reluctant to take car keys away, especially from a man.

Well, sorry, but I am very reluctant to watch more accidents, like one in my town where a mother and her daughter were killed by an old driver with dementia. And this will happen. Sometimes an older driver has simply driven away and never been seen again.

Past history of careful driving is no guarantee that drivers with dementia can make the right decisions to avoid killing someone. They drive the wrong way on freeways, drive through an open market killing fifteen people, etc. Please do *not* let your elder with dementia drive. Stand up and do what must be done. Make sure, at the same time, that you arrange alternative transportation for them.

Families have taken the keys, they have secretly disabled a vehicle, they have said the doctor insisted this person not drive, they have had the

DMV revoke a driving license. A determined person may still get round all this. One son sold his father's car and his father went out and bought another one.

It is hard to do this, but a good family does not let a demented person drive. If the moral side of this doesn't appeal to you, remember that a major lawsuit can come your way if you have allowed your father or mother to drive when they really were unable to manage the task.

Actually, women often give up driving when they feel they have become incapable, or often before then. It is really a bigger issue for the men. Remember that doctors in most states are now required to inform the DMV when someone has been diagnosed with dementia, and their license will be pulled.

Eating

Changes of eating patterns can occur in all elders and especially in those with Alzheimer's. To keep them eating well, make meals comforting and good – colorful foods, good protein, and old favorites all combined. Put the food on the plate, since often people can't serve themselves reasonable amounts of food. Observe what gets eaten and what doesn't, so you can satisfy their wants. Remember that a person with dementia probably can't give reliable information on what they want to eat.

Maybe this person wants certain foods that look tidy together, or items that must not touch each other on a plate. Maybe this person will eat everything on one side of the plate, and you will have to turn their plate so they can eat the food on the other side. All of these issues are dementia problems – maybe brain changes, memory issues, visual-spatial problems, small strokes. We never know for sure, and it doesn't really matter.

Just respect food idiosyncrasies. Don't mix things together if this person doesn't want that. Children often have the same feelings, so maybe this is a return to primal functioning. Our main goal is to keep good nutrition in this person's life. We might need to make more and smaller meals each day. Just experiment and find what works.

Sugar-hunger seems to be common in dementia. Caregivers report that their elder will happily eat six ice-cream bars at a time, or will secretly raid the freezer to sneak them out. High amounts of sugar are probably not very desirable for any elder, let alone those with diabetes.

Studies have shown that people with dementia use up about four thousand calories a day, a total that the average construction worker might use while doing roadwork. This is the result of brain function being always in struggle. I have been told by people with early dementia that they are exhausted from trying to keep on track all the time. We must assume this is true for those who can't communicate this so well. This constant brain activity probably causes the sugar-hunger. Studies have shown that people, even with late-stage dementia, have more dreams per night than those without, so there is always a lot of brain activity going on.

However, there may also be something different going on which you can help with. As mentioned earlier, all elders have a reduced number of digestive enzymes available to process food. This means that essential nutrients cannot be distributed around the body as needed. Starved of necessary complex sugars, brain functioning struggles. It may be that elders have a sugar-hunger because the brain is crying out for these complex sugars – which, of course, are not available from ice cream bars.

It is always worthwhile to add a full-spectrum enzyme capsule to daily medications, with your doctor's approval. We have found that mental acuity increases, sometimes markedly, in an elder with dementia once digestive enzymes are added.

Hoarding

It is quite common for people to hoard things – food stashed in drawers, quantities of canned goods, even a hidden collection of all the soft toys in the house. Some people hoard banknotes or other valuables. For some, this is a reaction to their fears that they are losing things of value – such as their memory and their former life. Others will be seeking a sense of security from hoarding. And others – well, they might just want a big old bundle of bears tucked away under their pillow.

Inappropriateness

When a person has dementia, everyone else better get ready to deal with some embarrassing moments. Since they'll happen anyway, I suggest you enjoy them. A couple of my favorites came from the time when I was looking after Hannah in Berkeley.

Once, while having coffee in a Berkeley coffee shop, Hannah took out her teeth and casually washed them in her cup of coffee, watched with shock by the woman at the next table. Another time we were forced to share a table with two other women, both of them quite plump. Hannah looked around cheerfully and said, "Well, I can only say that everybody..." and here she paused for a moment and the two women looked at her with polite interest, "everybody is much too fat!" I had to explain to our indignant tablemates that Hannah had Alzheimer's and did not really mean to be offensive.

People often express fears that their elder with dementia might be sexually inappropriate, but this is usually based upon behaviors like a woman pulling up her underwear in view of others, a man failing to zip his pants, or unzipping them to urinate in a nearby waste bin. All of these are ways in which a child might be inappropriate until trained, and they signal the loss of recognition of polite and appropriate behaviors.

Incontinence

This is the big fear of families dealing with dementia. It is actually at the big divide between home care and facility care and is the single biggest reason families seek facility care for their member.

Here is the good news – in dementia, there is nothing inevitable about incontinence. Only about ten percent of people with Alzheimer's become incontinent, that is, due to genuine loss of bodily control. For the rest, the issue is really a failure to remember where the bathroom is and maybe what it's for, or being unable to recognize internal signals that warn them their body is ready for elimination of waste products.

A program of a once-an-hour trip to the bathroom will help. You may have to accompany the person to the bathroom, and you would be very wise to learn the normal elimination habits and work with them. Most people have a regular pattern of bowel movements. After breakfast or after lunch are typical and you can work with this.

If your elder says, "Oh, I don't need to," make a calm suggestion but don't give orders. People with dementia find it hard to oppose suggestions, because that requires good rationality skills, which they no longer have. However, they can lock solid against orders.

"Well, let's try anyway, because we're going to eat soon," you might say.

Family members often find it very hard to understand these changes in elders, but that is because they have forgotten how we all have to learn about using the toilet when we are toddlers. Instead, they are caught up in a sense of shame on behalf of their oblivious elder, which is a common projection, but not especially useful.

As we age, we may forget many things we learned if we have dementia. We no longer know what a certain bodily feeling is trying to tell us. It is part of our loss of cognitive ability. This is where a regular bathroom schedule helps. It helps your elder and it will help you.

Part of our trouble is our societal attitudes about urine and feces. We certainly don't want to deal with our parent's feces in any form and one solution for incontinence dread is preparation. Have protective gloves, antiseptic wipes, plenty of toilet paper, and protective underwear available – masks, too, if you want to.

In my household, we always make jokes about this sometimes messy process, though not within earshot of the person concerned.

"Oh my goodness, call in the HazMat team!" we'll say to each other and that helps us cope better. Or we speculate about whether we could just get a giant cat tray.

When we had one resident with special elimination issues, we took to categorizing the results like fires. A good day was just a two-alarm deposit, a worse day a five-alarm. Not so tasteful, I realize, but we all amuse ourselves as best we can when care life gets stressful.

One gentleman we knew had been a zookeeper and he used animals to categorize the amount of diarrhea his poor wife eliminated. "Enough to kill an elephant," he'd report sometimes, and we would commiserate.

If someone has become incontinent and needs protective underwear, confiscate all other underwear so they have to use medical pull-ups. No one feels great about these transitions because they often feel a bit ashamed, as if they were little children wearing diapers. They feel it's somehow their fault, as if they should just control themselves better, not be like babies.

Best tackle this straightforwardly. Talk about it in a very matter-of-fact manner and you can dissipate this shame easily.

"You know, Charles," I said to one gentleman, "Most older people use these things. It's a medical problem that causes the troubles. It's not your fault. It's your kidneys' fault. No one will ever know you're wearing these. Even if you had an accident, no one would know about that either. So, you'll actually feel much more relaxed about going out."

The other concern with possible incontinence is the protection of furniture, mattresses, armchairs, and so on. You can often make do cheaply by using plastic bags or sheeting rather than those very expensive medical sheets and covers, though you may be able to get those cheaply through your doctor's prescription. Be sure to ask. Most people adjust surprisingly fast to this. Many people who dreaded this moment find it's not so bad, as long as you have all the equipment ready.

One caregiver always told me that was when he'd put his wife into a care home, but when she did become incontinent, he found he could manage because of all the helpful equipment available these days. That includes a big-enough bathroom garbage can so you can instantly throw messy objects in there.

Should someone suddenly develop urinary incontinence, be sure to ask your doctor to arrange a urinalysis, as it is very likely that an infection has occurred. By the way, when a person with dementia gets a urinary tract infection, the dementia can suddenly appear to be much worse.

Memory Problems

This is at the heart of dementia and is usually the first major sign of illness. Some age-related memory issues are normal – such as forgetting appointments; looking for misplaced wallets, glasses and keys; being unable to recall a name and having it come to memory later.

These things are normal and may partly be due to lack of concentration, not paying attention to what we do, and maybe being out of the habit of brain-learning. This is a benign age-related memory issue. Almost everyone in their early sixties begins to experience this problem.

However, major memory problems, such as being unable to find a parked car, unable to find the way home, or having a complete memory blank-out so that you can't remember what you were going to do or where you are, are a sign of something more malignant. Paying the same bill over and over, or not at all, repetitive phone calls, confusion about daytime routines – these are alarming. By the time a person has been diagnosed with dementia, these problems will undoubtedly have increased greatly.

It is very important, by the way, that the family itself does not "diagnose" the problem. A person must have the full Alzheimer's work-up before diagnosis can be made. That is because many conditions look like what we think of as Alzheimer's. No diagnosis is made on appearance or guessing. Among those other frequent conditions are depression, small strokes, tumors, liver problems, lack of oxygen to the brain, cancer, and nutritional deprivation. Then there's over-medicating, alcoholism, and more. A full work-up with all the tests, radiography, examinations, and medical and social history must be done before any diagnosis can be made.

Once you know a person has dementia, you can either accept memory problems, work with them, or fight them. Accepting them is good and working with them is better. Knowing a person will forget the daily routine, you can write it up on a wall calendar or outline it on a blackboard or whiteboard. You can label cupboards. You can call at appropriate times with reminders. Probably all of these things will work for a while. Ultimately, maybe none of them will work, and this is another thing to accept and let go of. Each person does dementia in his or her own way and the memory issues are very individual, too. Learn just what form they take in your elder, make a plan accordingly, and don't worry about it.

Paranoia

Psychiatric jargon does not belong in the behavioral descriptions of people with dementia. This is because people with dementia are not mentally ill. They have organic brain problems that impair memory and logic processes. When we apply the jargon of the psychiatrist to the world of dementia, we depersonalize people and are less inclined to pay attention to what is really going on. This means we resist getting to know people as they are with dementia, and we are also in serious danger of ignoring their needs.

People with dementia do not have paranoia. They are rightly afraid because they are no longer protected by their memory and they are losing the capacity to run their own lives. Imagine that going on in your life and see how secure you feel.

Here is more psychiatric jargon that doesn't belong in dementia:

- Combative – describes a reaction to scary events or treatment. It means a caregiver, or someone else, has frightened this person by their behavior. Being invasive or loud or acting in a way this person cannot comprehend might all bring about violent reactions. Sometimes, as in the case of veterans, the real issue might be post-traumatic stress reactions involving flashbacks. This is not a dementia issue but may manifest in a person with dementia, especially at night. It really requires special intervention from a health professional.

- Perseveration – means saying the same stuff over and over. That's because nobody listened the first thirty-five times to what was actually being said.

- Confabulating – means making up stories to fill the information gaps in the brain's memory of what's going on in one's life. It doesn't mean lying.

Repetition

This can apply to behaviors, speech, stories, questions, or physical actions. It happens because short-term memory loss means no information is retained. However, it continues because of the way this person feels emotionally. It means there are needs not being addressed by caregivers. If we listen hard to the sub-text of any vocal repetition, we can often make excellent intuitive guesses about what the real issue is.

For example, if your mother asks over and over, "When is my mother coming home?" you can guess she needs to be mothered in order to feel safe and loved. You can divert the question by offering her something she might like to eat or helping her do something that makes her feel more secure. You can simply wrap your arms around her.

Sometimes a person will do the same action, over and over. One woman on the Oregon coast had several cats and dogs and fed them multiple times each day. She largely spent her day this way. I watched her carry helpings of food from the various food bags and deliver them to the dishes. This provided her with an occupation and the feeling that she was being useful and helpful to the animals she loved so much.

She had been a nurse for much of her life. Now her pets offered a way to nurture and care for others. The only downsides were the expense for the food and having three fat dogs. That seemed to me to be a fair trade for the pleasure and purposeful satisfaction this gave her.

It is very useful to examine any repetitive behavior using the Three-Point-Plan described earlier that I finally devised after years of looking at the problem behaviors of dementia. Try it and see if this formula works for you.

In the case of repetitive speech, if you can't divert or satisfy this person, then use the time-honored non-comment of parents everywhere – "Uh-huh." Choose not to be annoyed. Repetitive behaviors are due to illness and are just one more thing this person can't control.

One family was being driven to distraction by their mother's constant repetition of "When is Daddy coming home?" So they decided to start running a betting pool on how many times she would say this. They kept count, made their bets, and each day the nearest guess won ten dollars for that family member. It was, they said, the most fun they'd had with Mom for at least a year. They were not making fun of her. They were making fun for themselves to change the energy of frustration which otherwise would have built up. It worked.

Use your own ingenuity to make difficult repetition bearable. It can't be stopped, so try to have fun. Most of all, choose *not* to take it personally. It is loss of memory that makes a person repeat the same thing over and over, but it is the need of the person that shapes exactly what that repetition is. Those are the only two things you need to remember.

Rummaging

Searching through drawers, cupboards, closets, the china cabinet, handbags – this is normal in dementia. It is due to the disease, of course, but it may also represent a way of trying to deal with fear and loss.

This elder wants something to do, is anxious and upset, and may be feeling that just finding some lost thing will provide an answer. The best thing to do is either re-direct that energy into a different activity, if you can, or let it go. No point in driving yourself crazy about it. If there are things of yours you don't want messed with, then lock that particular access or move your items to a more secure hiding place.

Just understand that this is a very confused person's way of trying to make sense of a life which has become hopelessly senseless. If you can distract or find other activities for this person, great. If not, then nurture in yourself an ability to not focus on what can't be changed.

I'm a big believer in amusing oneself to get through a caregiver day. I would put a lot more interesting things into the drawers – table tennis balls, small cat-toy mice, Hershey's kisses, anything I could buy cheaply in large quantities that would fit into drawers.

Sun-Downing

This is one of the biggest problem issues in caregiving. Yet it is also one of the most informative and profound parts of a demented person's day. It is a recurrent time of agitation, upset, anger, neediness – any form of emotional overload. It happens nearly every day at more or less the same time. It is called sun-downing because it usually happens at the end of the afternoon.

It can start around 2 p.m. for some people and not until 6 p.m. for others. It typically continues for about two hours. Sun-downing is especially difficult for caregivers because of the agitation which usually accompanies it. This agitation is very contagious and caregivers are easily swept up into it.

However, you can simply stay calm, knowing that being agitated doesn't actually do your mother any harm and the agitation will pass. Often, during this time of agitation, you might learn something very real about this person's feelings. Commonly, while sun-downing, people accurately pinpoint their sorrows, their feelings of loneliness and uselessness, and the loss of love in their lives.

This is often echoed by the actual form sun-downing takes. Some want to go home to their parents' house, while others insist that their children are expecting them home to cook dinner. People refer to the things they did when they were useful, needed, loved, safe, and occupying the very center of their lives. Their theme has real and deep meaning, even if their calendar sense is inaccurate.

I once watched a ninety-one-year-old Italian resident in a care facility insisting that she had to catch a bus and go home. It was 4 p.m. She said to the staff nurse, "Can you show me where the bus stop is?"

The nurse tried to argue her out of it, using rational approaches. She showed her a current calendar and the daily newspaper, pointing out the dates, proving that her sons in their seventies were not coming home from school to dinner with Mom.

Finally, the old Italian woman, with tears in her eyes and her hand on her breast, said, "I can see what you're telling me, and I see it's right. But I can only tell you that in here," and she patted her heart, "I have two little boys who need me."

It was the clearest explanation of the dilemmas of sun-downing I have ever seen. While most sun-downing lasts for about two hours, some caregivers say that they know people who spend all night sun-downing. That means someone they know is active, frantic, and agitated all night long. My suggestion in such cases is that the family gets a new diagnosis.

In the few cases I have known of such people, they have, in fact, been afflicted by lifelong, undiagnosed mental illnesses of various kinds. Families often do not recognize mental illness in their own parents, especially their mothers. Mother is simply who she is – difficult or quirky or with anger-management problems.

However, barely controlled mental illness often gets out of control in old age. The person no longer has the energy or capacity to contain it, and this is what we sometimes see in the most disturbed people in dementia-care facilities. They are known as dual-diagnosis residents, because you can be both mentally ill and have dementia. Given that the elderly mentally ill can be very difficult and bizarre, it is important for families to seek extra help for them. Otherwise, they may be abused in care facilities because of their difficult behaviors.

It can be possible to bring dementia-only sun-downing under better control. Since we don't know for sure what causes it, we need to take a multi-channel approach to deal with it. Assume that it is partly due to hunger, thirst, and weariness, plus whatever emotional issues are at work. About two hours before your elder usually starts sun-downing, offer a small snack and a fruit drink, plus some water.

Also make sure that an after-lunch nap has been taken. My experience does not suggest that small naps use up sleep potential at night. In fact, elders with dementia are often exhausted for much of their day. So much confusion going on in their minds really uses up a lot of energy.

Have an action plan ready for the sun-downing time – anything that works, from a favorite DVD on TV, looking through a family photo album together, taking a drive, dancing the tango, whatever. The key words are divert, persuade, bribe, and re-direct, not with words but with the actions you undertake. If none of this works, just sit down and let it be. Pick up a book and read for a while, or turn on Oprah. By the way, everyone with dementia loves to watch *Oprah, Wheel of Fortune, Jeopardy, CNN*, and *Animal Planet*. Agitation never killed anyone and when it's over, for someone with dementia, it's over. So, at worst, sit it out.

Wandering

This is called "walking" when we do it but "wandering" when people with dementia do it. It is useful to remember just how this restriction could be disturbing to someone who feels the need to get out and move. People self-medicate their anxiety by walking. This is the major reason why people with dementia do this. Sometimes it is also a very literal way of going to look for their lost life.

Although it is certainly important to keep someone safe, we need to include a walking program in the life of someone who really likes and needs to do this. If you can't take this person walking, make a plan so that someone else does. Not many people are as lucky as the two branches of one family who arranged for Mom to walk back and forth between their two homes. She did, and she never got lost.

You, on the other hand, must make sure that your elder has usable I.D. on his or her person. Not in a handbag, which can be lost, nor in a wallet, which can be stolen. Use a wrist or ankle for this I.D., or put it round the neck like a military dog tag. At the very least it needs to say "MEMORY-IMPAIRED" and list your phone number.

The other important part of the wanderer's care plan is to have your house secured so no one can leave in the middle of the night, or even in the daytime, without you knowing it. You also need to have a photo ready for police in case you do lose your elder. Don't delay doing this on the grounds that your elder has never gone out alone before. There can always be a first time, and some people never return alive from that one-time outing.

House security need not be expensive. It can be cheap and ingenious. Use those little sets of door alarms, very inexpensive and easy to put up, with a choice of chimes. Some people like a string of little bells on the door that jingle loudly enough to warn everyone someone's sneaking out. We also like those hinged door-blockers that prevent a door being pulled open. Place them at the top and high up on the side where most people with dementia never think of looking. All doors, and gateways as well, need to be secured in some practical way.

There is Meaning in Dementia Nonsense

Let me show you exactly how Alzheimer's logic works. That way, you might usefully rack your own brains when confronted by bizarre behaviors to find the essential truth inside the behavior. Because, I can promise you, it is always there. Use the eyes of your heart to see, not your brain.

I used to care for an elder who lived on the Oregon coast, in a little house next to her daughter's cottage. Stevie was eighty-three years old and a delightful human being. Although she had apparently been an anxious and rather stern perfectionist earlier in her life, she had become a joyful, rather pixie-like woman delighted with her daily routine. She appreciated living.

Once when I made lunch for us both, she said happily, "I'm enjoying this food so much my teeth are singing!"

Stevie loved her pets – her three indoor cats, her three indoor dogs, and her five garage cats. She is the woman mentioned above who patrolled from one food bowl to another, making sure that each bowl was full at all times. Consequently, she had a collection of rather portly pets, but she loved to feel that she was looking after their needs.

Oregon coast winter nights get damp, cold, and rainy and her daughter bought a nice new electric blanket for Stevie. The next morning, when I turned up for work, I found the daughter almost vibrating with rage and Stevie standing with her head hanging down. Her daughter slammed angrily out of the house and, after her daughter had left, I turned to Stevie.

"Is something wrong?" I asked.

Stevie whispered to me, "She's mad at me." I knew who "she" was.

"Why?" I whispered back.

Stevie then told me why her daughter was so mad at her and it's a very charming story.

The previous night had been the first really chilly, raw night of the winter and she used her new electric blanket for the first time. As soon as she was in bed, warm and cozy under her blanket, she began to worry about all her pets and whether they would be warm enough, like her.

So she got up, fetched a pair of scissors and, having first unplugged the blanket – thank goodness – carefully cut it up into large squares which she then distributed to the pets, tucking one square under each cat or dog to keep it warm.

I loved Stevie for doing this and I also love that this is the perfect example of Alzheimer's logic, which always has some vital piece of rationality missing. Stevie did not do this because she was crazy. She did it because she loved her pets and wanted them to be as comfortable as she was, but had forgotten the real workings of an electric blanket. This is a story of what great souls do when they get Alzheimer's.

A LIFE IN ALZHEIMER'S LAND

Hannah's life had been dramatic in many ways. She had a mother who never nurtured her.

"She lay in bed eating chocolates and crying!" she told me once with disgust.

She loved her father. "A wonderful, wonderful man!" she smiled.

They lived in Dresden, a city rich in culture and fabulously beautiful – a beauty which was firebombed into rubble in the Second World War. Their families were prosperous Jews. Her father owned a pharmacy business. Hannah herself had a successful career as an actress until the Nazis came to power. She was the first actress in Germany to play the part of St. Joan in the Bernard Shaw play. Once the Nazis were in power, however, Jews could no longer act on the public stage.

She met and married an ambitious, young, Polish physician, also a Jew. In 1938, she and her husband came as refugees to America. Hannah's beloved father could come with them, on one condition – that he leave his wife behind. Hannah, her father, and her husband all survived. Her mother vanished into concentration camp dust, with no one in the family knowing what camp she was taken to. Everyone else in the family died in the concentration camps as well.

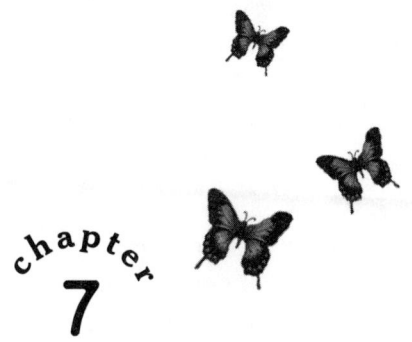

Help From Nature

Be hopeful. Medical research into Alzheimer's represents the spending of millions of funding dollars. There are many promising lines of development, including new explorations of brain chemistry processes in the normal working of the human brain, about which we have known surprisingly little. Alzheimer's is probably now the most-researched illness on the planet. This is very good news for everyone undertaking the Alzheimer's journey, either as a caregiver, family member, or as someone who actually has this dementia.

So be very, very hopeful. Remember that when diabetes research was being carried out in 1921, insulin was announced as a successful treatment. Families everywhere knew they had been saved. Literally overnight, diabetes moved from being a terminal illness to a health condition that could be controlled by use of insulin.

There is no reason why Alzheimer's researchers could not find a similar solution for control of dementia. Always hold that hope. There is a continuing series of experimental drugs and research programs going on now, each one hoping to have the key to slowing or even overcoming Alzheimer's. Most people diagnosed as having a dementia of the Alzheimer's type will be offered opportunities to become part of such research. When offered the chance to become part of an experimental program, think it through carefully. Read all the information available on the proposed research before making a decision about participation, including anything you can find out about possible negative side effects. It is often better to be part of the second research year than the first, because at that point the side effects will be more fully known. But it is always your own decision.

People with dementia can be more easily compromised by drug effects. That said, it is entirely a family's own decision. Some people feel enhanced by becoming part of research that might bring a breakthrough, for others even if not for themselves, and this is noble motivation.

As a family member or caregiver, be very watchful of any possible side effects. Intervene if you see enough negative effects to compromise the daily comfort of the person you care for. Make your own decision and be confident of your own observations, because you *are* the on-the-spot expert on your own elder. You are the gatekeeper who keeps that person safe. Contributing to human medical development is wonderful, but losing life quality in the process should not be part of that.

Some families have reported undue pressure from researchers to continue in experimental research when they feel they already see adverse side effects. This should be an immediate warning not to continue, since it means those researchers are willing to risk participants' well-being for their own ends. Use your personal judgment and don't let your family member be compromised. Be judicious about programs that interfere with normal life or disrupt a routine that is a comfort to you or your elder.

Remember Alzheimer's is a slow process, so you probably won't lose so very much by letting others be in the first ranks while you wait for the side effects to emerge. If a treatment shows great promise, you will hear about it soon enough.

When you read about new Alzheimer's treatments in the newspaper, do your own due diligence and research further. You'll find out that this is not necessarily the magic bullet or that it is not even being tested solely on people with a diagnosis of Alzheimer's. In the past thirty years, many such temporary excitements have arisen. Remember the hype about aluminum? The basic issue is that Alzheimer's and similar dementias represent a long cascade of developments. Many of the researchers are finding little bits of the process. The complexity of brain chemistry makes research even more demanding.

When you add factors seldom touched upon by researchers – that human beings live long, complex lives full of influences, events, and outcomes and that possibly the key to dementia might be in some of these – you can see that one small pill may not always be the answer.

However, everything good in your own health regime will always be positive for you. Eat right, sleep fully, walk or exercise appropriately, have a pet, listen to music, and so on – all these things are good for you and your elder. The good things of life remain important and research demonstrates they have very positive effects on people with dementia and their caregivers.

When it comes to natural remedies, be as cautious about them as you are about commercially processed drugs. Any time you read that some new product, discovery, tree, or herb heals more than one major illness, be dubious. If they are touted to heal ten, be downright disbelieving, but try them anyway if you want to.

In general, if you want to know about the long-term healing capacity of herbs, spices, or other plants, look to the medical traditions of countries with a long written history of observation of results from using such plants. Look at traditional Chinese medicine, with its first written medical text dating from three thousand years ago, *The Yellow Emperor's Classic of Internal Medicine.*

Think it's all ancient superstition? Think again. Chinese traditional medicine was treating diabetes, called "the thirsting sickness," in 200 AD using the pancreas of pigs for insulin.

It was also treating asthma at that time with the ephedra plant (ephedrine), which is still the basic ingredient in modern Western asthma treatment.

Look also at Ayurvedic medicine, the traditional medicine of India. Their spices and herbs are currently being researched by Western medical researchers who are finding that they actually do what traditional Ayurvedic doctors use them to do – treat hepatitis, blood pressure, cancer, and so on. Take a look at homeopathy, a treatment system used in the West for over two hundred years and offering treatments that have no side effects, are very cheap, and may or may not help.

In all of these systems, you can try remedies for little cost that have few or no side effects, so find out for yourself if they seem to help. Be pro-active. Remember that modern medicine has done very little to successfully help those with dementia, so you are free to try. Just don't fall for schemes or silver bullets, or pay a lot. Really, if there were a secret remedy for Alzheimer's that provided an overnight cure, the whole world would know by now. So don't run in panicked hope even to the other side of the USA, let alone to Europe or Asia.

That said, here are some possible helpers for you. They are cheap and easily found on the Internet or in your local health food or produce store, so go for it.

Natural Remedies

Anything harmless that will boost the immune system is helpful, since there is a good possibility that what we call Alzheimer's might in fact be an age-related autoimmune disease. Even if it isn't, immune boosters are always helpful.

Increasingly research offers some very useful information on which nutrients, vitamins, herbs, and minerals can help support brain function. This list is by no means comprehensive but will get you started. Keep checking on the latest information and immediately cut out relevant articles.

In all cases of nutritional and herbal supplementation, either follow printed directions or ask your doctor's advice for dosage. Also, check with reliable online resources. (See the Resources section.) You can't always rely on the information on websites aimed at getting you to buy their product, so always do your own research.

Cat's claw is a tropical vine that has been medicinally used in South America and Asia and has been found to reduce blood pressure, increase circulation, reduce cholesterol, and support the immune system. Vascular deficiency is what lessens the flow of blood to the brain, so something that increases such circulation and is also an immune booster may be helpful. It comes in capsules, tea, and extract form.

Coenzyme Q – The Mayo Clinic states that this is naturally occurring in the human body and helps the basic functioning of cells and supports the immune system. Since its presence decreases with age, some researchers question whether this decrease is also part of the picture of dementia. It has been shown to decrease blood pressure and macular degeneration, and taking it is thought to increase oxygen supply to the brain. It protects cells, supports cardiovascular processes, and also has strong antioxidant powers. Some medical researchers regard it as potentially very helpful for elders whose natural antioxidant resources are being reduced by age. Heart specialists are increasingly exploring its ability to dramatically improve heart health.

Digestive enzymes – Since seeing the positive results of these, I now recommend them to all elders. Brain health depends upon all the benefits of your food reaching the brain and body. Without sufficient digestive enzymes, this does not happen.

There are many brands of digestive enzymes but we have found the best to be Enzymedica's Digest Gold. It has fifteen different enzymes in it and can be found online at bargain prices.

Garlic – There are many good things about garlic – it cleans your blood of cholesterol, reduces inflammation in the body, and promotes heart health. Poor heart function lowers oxygen supply to the brain and is connected with brain inflammation. If you don't like actual garlic, you can take no-odor garlic pills.

Ginkgo biloba – The oldest species of tree still living, with a two-hundred-million-year ancestry, has leaves long used for medicinal purposes in traditional Chinese medicine, treating asthma and other respiratory conditions. Modern research shows it to be a vascular enhancer, bringing more blood flow to the brain and increasing the uptake of glucose by brain cells. It is also showing ability to improve the transmission of nerve signals, may build antioxidant power in the body and brain, and could possibly prove to be helpful in fighting macular degeneration.

This is still being researched but many users report experiencing short-term memory improvement, and it has become a standard in brain-function herbal formulas. The recommended extract or pill is composed of twenty-four percent Ginkgo flavone glycosides and six percent terpene lactones.

Ginkgo is also a blood thinner, so be sure to let your doctor know you are taking it, especially if you are going to undergo a surgical procedure of any kind.

Ginseng – Siberian ginseng and American ginseng are both considered to be helpful in improving vascular supply to the brain, but should be used very carefully by those with high blood pressure. Ask your doctor's advice on this.

Homeopathy – Useful in memory issues and seems to hold the dementia at a plateau for an unusual length of time, at least in some cases. Homeopathic remedies are available in many health food stores and food co-ops, but are often cheaper online. (See Resources section.) Best choices for good homeopathic supplies are Boiron or Standard.

Using the homeopathic bible, *Boericke's Materia Medica*, you can look up suggested remedies for particular conditions. Since it predates the term Alzheimer's disease, you can look under behavior symptoms to find suggested remedies. In homeopathy, there are eight direct remedies for different kinds of memory problems and different kinds of people. The following are homeopathically-prepared remedies, not the raw herb or mineral:

1. **Anacardium:** for loss of memory or weak memory in a person with digestive problems, who likes to walk a lot, has heart palpitations, skin problems, and suffers from sleeplessness

2. **Sulphur:** for memory loss associated with names and words in the person who typically is irritable and depressed, has inflamed eyes, drinks much and eats little, wants windows open, has rheumatism, and likes warm, dry weather

3. **Baryta carb:** for memory problems that seem like absent-mindedness in a depressed moody person with hair loss, deafness, catches colds easily, has pains in feet, and twitches in sleep

4. **Zinc:** for memory problems in a person who seems sleepy and lethargic as if it were hard to think, has bleeding gums, watering eyes, heartburn from sweet foods, constipation, asthmatic bronchitis, and night sweats

5. **Cocculus:** for memory problems associated with anxiety and distraction in a person who suffers migraines, stomach upsets, constant drowsiness, and frequent low fevers

6. **Digitalis:** for memory problems associated with being unable to think things through logically in a person having eye problems, liver problems, heart palpitations, and swelling of hands and feet

7. **Ethusa cynapium:** for memory problems associated with being unable to concentrate in a person with restlessness and anxiety, lactose intolerance, dry mouth, constipation, difficulty breathing, and walks with clenched hands

8. **Rhododendron:** for memory problems associated with losing trains of thought while talking in a person with hearing problems that improve in the morning, frequent breathlessness, and widespread arthritis

Homeopathic remedies look like little sugar pills and the suggested dose is usually four pills four times a day. Don't touch them with your fingers; shake them into the bottle cap and drop them under your tongue and let them dissolve there. They come in many different doses and unless you get direct advice from a homeopathic MD, which is recommended, buy the 3X or 6X strength. There are no bad side effects from homeopathy and it is cheap. Try it and keep notes on what you observe. Trust your own research and – no, Virginia – it's not necessary to believe in it.

Horse-chestnut extract is a powerful anti-inflammatory that has many antioxidant qualities and contains a substance called aescin, which strengthens and repairs veins and capillaries. You should look for extract strength with fifteen to twenty percent aescin and a supplement dosage of at least 50 mg. It complicates the use of blood thinners, so you must tell your doctor if you're taking this plant extract.

Huperzine A is a naturally occurring alkaloid found in the plant extracts of the fir moss *Huperzia serrata*. Researchers in China, Europe, and the United States are looking into its neuro-protective properties and the National Institute of Health is in the secondary stages of double-blind studies. There is a lot of hope about the possible usefulness of this alkaloid in aiding and supporting brain function. Some people report allergic reactions to the liquid extract, which seem less frequent from the capsule form. Huperzine is also included in capsule form in a number of brain formulas.

Kava-Kava is a plant from the South Sea Islands with the property of calming without causing lack of mental clarity. It is usually available in capsule or liquid extract and is marketed as a remedy for insomnia, anxiety, and stress.

L-arginine is an amino acid which limited research has shown to be a possible help in increasing oxygen supply to the brain.

Lavender essential oil – Wonderful to use around the house to calm, cheer, and support emotional well-being. You can diffuse it throughout the day and, used nightly in the bedroom, it can help restless people to sleep. This can also be used during typical sun-downing time and has been well documented as being able to help reduce agitation.

I have recommended its use in care facilities with the result that sun-downing behaviors become much calmer and less agitated than usual. Always get pure essential oil, not chemical fragrances which do not have the same benefits. You can put a drop directly on the skin, one on each side of the neck, which allows the aroma to rise directly towards the person's nose.

Lemon balm essential oil – Also improves memory and lifts the spirits.

Lemon essential oil – When diffused or sprayed in a room, it both energizes and elevates mood.

Passionflower, despite its name, is actually an herbal sleep-aide. It is available as a tea, a liquid extract, or in capsule form. It helps relax and calm, leading to a good night's sleep.

Phosphatidylserine is a naturally occurring chemical, which provides nutritional support for brain function and which brain researchers consider possibly helpful in Alzheimer's or similar dementias.

Rosemary essential oil – Traditionally associated with memory in herbal lore, it has been tested by the Arizona Office of Agriculture on elders and found to raise memory function as well as Cognex. It is easy to use around the house in a diffuser or sprayed as a rosemary oil/water mixture (4 oz. spring water, 30 drops of rosemary essential oil).

Valerian is a well-established herbal remedy used for stress and insomnia. It helps a person sleep without setting up a dependency or carrying over into the day as a hangover. Used throughout the day, it is calming without being tranquillizing. It can be used in tea form, capsule, and liquid extract. A person with dementia could use it, as could a stressed caregiver, and it might help with nighttime restlessness.

Vinpocetine is a chemical derived from the lesser periwinkle plant, and researchers are looking at its effects on brain function, memory improvement, and increased vascular supply to the brain. It is considered promising but with too little official research done yet. You might want to use it in an already established commercial brain formula since the plant itself has some toxic side effects, which a commercial formula is unlikely to have.

Vitamins – Everyone knows by now that extra vitamins are a good idea in our world of over-processed food. However, even in the vitamin world, there is a struggle over what exactly is the right mix and dosage. Guidelines vary as new information comes up, and it is a good idea to follow the recommendations of a doctor more in tune with the issues, such as Andrew Weil, Earl Mindell, and others.

We know for sure that certain vitamin deficiencies in themselves cause dementia and also reduce elder health in other ways. Vitamin B deficiencies are associated with reversible dementia and one of the reasons is that the B vitamins are not stored for long in the body. Elders typically may not be replenishing them in their food. B12, folic acid, and niacin deficiencies are all associated with reversible dementia and a blood test can reveal these deficiencies. Supplemental B complex, B12, and folic acid are a great idea for elders, whether or not dementia is present. Vitamin E (400 - 800 IU per day) and vitamin C (1,000 mg three times per day) are recommended by the University of Maryland Medical Center to be taken together as powerful antioxidant support for the brain.

Zinc – Up to 50 mg a day is recommended for immune system support and possible memory improvement.

Stress-Busters

As a caregiver, you will undoubtedly need some handy stress-reduction activities to keep you nice, and you may find that your elder will also enjoy some of these. For example, in one of my care homes we had a yoga teacher come twice a week and all the residents enjoyed following along with her. They could not have remembered what to do, left to themselves, but they were very happy to do it under her leadership. I strongly recommend either yoga or Tai Chi for caregivers because both are ancient forms of exercise based upon supporting harmony and the good flow of energy in the body.

If you can't find or can't get out to classes, there are many DVDs for home study. You don't need a special space for these disciplines and can actually do many of the exercises in your own living room, following your DVD instructor. You can buy these items at bargain prices on eBay and Amazon.com. If your income does not allow you to purchase them even at reduced prices, then check with your local library. I'll bet you'll find them there, too.

Chi Kung was developed within the Taoist tradition of ancient China. It is a very slow form of movement, breath work, and meditation. It works the entire energy system of the body in a gentle, slow, yet powerful way to bring peace, health, and harmony to the whole being. In China today, elders are required to do Tai Chi or Chi Kung before they can have their meals at senior centers. It is the country's commitment to keeping the elderly healthy. It is suitable for people of all ages, from young to ancient. Elders unused to standing can do Chi Kung very well whilst seated in a chair and doing the range of movements very gently.

Swimming provides low physical stress and is a very good exercise for people of all ages. Elders with dementia have a range of responses to this activity. It's worth a try if someone had formerly been a person who enjoyed swimming. Not specially recommended as a new experience for a person with dementia, but if you feel lucky...

Tai Chi is a wonderfully gentle yet thoroughly exercising series of stylized movements. Coming from ancient China, it is a slow workout for every muscle in the body, using breath and harmonious movement to bring the whole body into balance. It can be done seated in a chair and many elders with dementia really love to do this.

Walking is a great form of exercise for everyone, young and old.

Fortunately, many people with dementia are in fairly good physical condition and walking is interesting and calming for them. Avoid trying this on windy days – most elders with Alzheimer's are very sensitive to the wind and find it disturbing.

Yoga is a form of exercise which also enhances breathing, calmness, flexibility, overall well-being, and a sense of harmony. Developed in India three thousand years ago, you can find classes today in every town all over the United States, including at many churches, or you can find DVDs on eBay and Amazon.com.

Peaceful Pursuits

Aromatherapy baths are my personal favorite for deep relaxation – a nice hot bath with rose, lavender, or geranium essential oil at night; in the morning (not my best time of day), one of the citrus essential oils to wake me up.

Driving the car is not to be done by the person with dementia, of course, but going out in the car is great for caregivers and those they care for. It is soothing; the passing of the landscape usually seems to bring a lot of pleasure, and the rhythm and sound of a car seems as peaceful as it is for restless babies. Use this as a great diversion when one is needed – to change a mood, cheer someone up, or just bring something new into a day. Seat belts must be worn and doors must be locked, preferably with a child-lock installed.

Music is soothing for caregivers and the people they care for. As much as you may enjoy New Age meditative music, many elders don't. Go with the music enjoyed by your elder – Lawrence Welk, classic Country and Western, whatever.

Pets are great for caregivers and people with dementia. Many relationships are damaged or changed when a person has Alzheimer's, and many friends can become elusive out of fear or embarrassment. A cat or dog can be a great consolation, even for elders who have never enjoyed pets before, and pets are great for caregivers, too.

Meditation is not some fancy foreign thing that decent Christian people can't do. The contemplative side of Christianity is actually a centuries-old discipline, though all too seldom used these days. The point of meditation in all traditions is essentially the same: to bring peaceful quietness to the mind. The easiest way to do this is to sit quietly and breathe slowly and deeply. There are books, DVDs, and CDs to teach meditation from any tradition, including the body health and fitness tradition. Go for it. You'll be a much better caregiver – and a nicer person.

A LIFE IN ALZHEIMER'S LAND

As her father abandoned his wife, Hannah's husband seemed to have emotionally abandoned his wife and three sons. He died on vacation with his mistress at the age of fifty-four. Hannah's three sons also abandoned their mother in their own various ways. They tended to ignore her, were often angry that she was ill, and had few emotionally positive connections with her. However, they did enable her to be looked after at home by encouraging the team of informal and inexperienced caregivers that gathered around to care for her. It was a huge and surprisingly imaginative contribution to her welfare.

This was a difficult family, with complex emotional undercurrents, in which Hannah's children seemed unhappy. Obviously she must have played her own part in the past that created their tension-ridden present. As for Hannah herself, however, in some ways she had become a much simpler person. She was happy. Her needs were taken care of. She had people surrounding her whose sole focus was to create an environment in which she could maintain that state of happiness.

Her sons, with many more resources, seemed to have less. Perhaps that was why they often seemed angry with their mother. In my innocence, I had no idea how often this occurs in families dealing with dementia. Now I know better. It is often almost unbearable for children who have been ill nurtured by their parent to become ideal caregivers to that parent. If outsiders take on the job successfully, as they so often can, it is often equally painful for them.

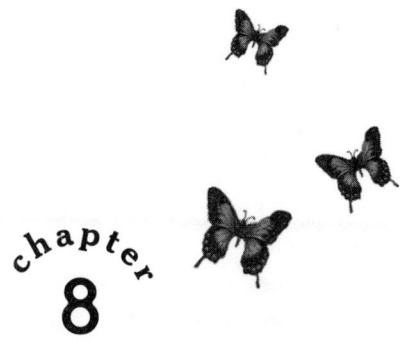

Forgiveness and Acceptance

Most people have problems being an Alzheimer's caregiver. It is certainly true that there is a lot to do and a lot to keep track of, plus there is the delicate management of a person who is your parent, your spouse, or otherwise familiar person in a different role.

However, there is a big elephant in the drawing room of Alzheimer's care and no one wants to talk about it. We shall talk about it, because it is essential to your own welfare that we do. While I totally understand that this situation is both hard for you and not what you wanted, so what? While I know that your mother, father, spouse, or brother is not the person you once knew, so what? While I get it that you suffer, *so what?*

I want to challenge those attitudes – the almost universal sorry-for-ourselves, pity for the person with Alzheimer's, appalled by its awfulness, blah, blah, blah. These may be the attitudes fully supported by our society. However, they are attitudes that kill. They get the person with dementia nowhere and they are going to drown you, as they have drowned many other caregivers.

When we let ourselves be washed over by this continuing sea of negativity, we suffer needlessly. Worse, we make the person we care for suffer needlessly. That's the bit that really bothers me. You have choices, but that person with dementia does not have that easy freedom you have.

They are trapped, within their disease condition *and* with you.

Don't both of you deserve better? Alzheimer's dementia is what it is – difficult and challenging, asking us to grow as we must. We need to develop a much more meditative state of mind about it all and we need to look deeper into ourselves as caregivers.

I was once at a care facility on the Oregon Coast, doing a training session for staff. After I finished, I went into the residents' lounge and sat down in an armchair. I was sitting near a cheerful, friendly man, and we chatted together in a sociable way. Clearly he had a lot of impairment in his thinking and memory, but he was eager to talk. After a while, the door of the lounge opened and a woman came in.

My new friend raised his hand and called out enthusiastically, "There she is! My angel! My darling!"

The woman came over and sat near him, scowling. Her husband got up to get her a cup of coffee and I said to her, "Your husband obviously loves you dearly."

"I hate it when he talks like that," she said grimly. "He was never like that. He was an engineer. He never talked in any kind of emotional way."

"Well, now he does," I said. "Sometimes that's what happens in this illness. People have losses but they also really open up their hearts more."

"I want the way he used to be," she insisted.

"I know," I answered, "but you have only one choice here. Either you move forward to where he is now, or you and he both stay alone and lonely. That other man you knew lived in a different time. This is the man who's here now. This is it."

Her painful dilemma is very common among those relating to a person changed by illness and is a constant issue in dementia. Many family relationships depend upon assumptions, roles, and unspoken expectations, certainly in marriage, especially a long marriage. Rules are important and illness brings change to the rules, especially since the one with dementia can no longer remember them.

Husbands get angry when elderly wives cannot carry out duties as housekeepers, cooks, and organizers. Wives become upset when something happens that literally changes the personality of their husbands. Adult children, too, struggle to establish a new kind of relationship with parents who now seem to need parents of their own.

You might think that these difficulties only happen in families which have had dissension and problems before, but that isn't necessarily so. I once had to help a new resident settle into a care home when her daughter brought her in. The new resident, a very charming elderly woman called Edie, was settled down on the sofa by her daughter, who was agitated and unhappy.

I took her daughter into the kitchen and made coffee for her.

"I'll make sure your mom is okay," I said. "Don't worry."

"I feel terrible about bringing her to somewhere like this!" she told me.

"I know. I understand," I assured her. "I'll be here to help her settle in and I'll be keeping a close eye on how she's doing. She'll probably do fine. There are other ladies for her to make friends with and I'll see she doesn't get too lonely."

What emerged from our conversation surprised me. She and her mother had been very close, she explained. Very close.

"I always felt that my mother was my best friend," she said tearfully. "We talked about everything. We read the same books and we'd talk about them. We went to concerts together."

She really did mean it when she described her mother as her best friend. They were very close and she had never married. She had her job and her mother and that made her life...until Alzheimer's came along.

"Now I just can't stand her!" she said. "I can't bear the way she's changed."

Eventually, the daughter went home to her now empty house and I went to spend time with her mother. By my standards, her mother was really not very impaired. She was friendly, easily engaged in conversation, and managed life graciously, with some impairment.

That daughter, like the engineer's wife, had left herself bereft and without any consolation for her loss. When people have dementia, our only choice is to move into the present where they are. The past has gone and with it the person they once were. If we refuse to move into their present, we lose both the past – because, after all, it has gone – and any possibility for the future. Then, yes, we are left with nothing.

The problem is that Alzheimer's represents everything that we as a society most fear. We fear becoming less than we are, losing our independence, losing our dignity, becoming like children, and having no power. We fear the loss of our very selves and we judge people with dementia as having lost their very selves.

Why does Alzheimer's alone affect us so deeply that we can scarcely bring ourselves to stand by our own relatives? Why are people with Alzheimer's so often deserted by friends? So pitied and feared by strangers? I believe it is because Alzheimer's strikes at the very heart of what so many human beings fear – to be unloved, unvalued, and seemingly undeserving of love. We will be unable to earn love if we have nothing to give.

And so many have already had such terrible lessons in how there really is not enough love for them, that to be a babe in human arms does not get us what we yearn for – loving acceptance, tenderness, and safety. It is that early lesson in the insufficiency of love that so distorts the way we look at Alzheimer's. It has skewed everything and we do not even recognize that our problem is what is inside our own hearts, not the disease affecting someone else.

So how do we help ourselves? We do it by coming back into relationship with this person. Instead of running, we sit beside this person and deal with our pain and our panic. This is the deepest and most profound way we heal ourselves and bring comfort to this person. It is really much simpler than people believe.

We can choose to feel differently. We can choose not to indulge ourselves in despair. We can choose not to be angry. We can choose to forgive instead. That, after all, is the real problem – that we blame the person with Alzheimer's for being ill.

I have actually had a granddaughter say of her grandmother, "If she'd taken better care of herself, this wouldn't have happened."

I said, as gently as I could (since her grandmother was a personal favorite of mine), "All kinds of people who took really good care of themselves have dementia. Healthy people who ate well and exercised, smart people with Nobel prizes, and silly neglectful people – they have all ended up with Alzheimer's."

And it's true. As hard as we try, we can't guarantee we won't get a bad disease. People die of lung cancer who never once smoked. People die of cirrhosis who never drank. There are diseases out there and statistically we get them. God doesn't hand them out like slices of poisoned cake. It happens. Things just happen. And sometimes they happen to you. Those who blame the sick person probably are terrified they too will end up stricken, so they try to create a blame scenario – she did this, so she got that. That would guarantee that people only got the diseases they deserved and, conversely, that if this person got that disease, it was because of personal behavior.

It would also mean that sick people don't deserve our love and that we can deal with the whole loss-sorrow-pity thing by avoiding it. Meanwhile, back in real life, grandmas get illnesses that their families don't know what to do with or about. And it hurts. That's the real issue, isn't it? Much easier to blame, point the finger, and be angry about diseases we fear than to look at our own fear and hurt.

Hidden inside all this, of course, is a part we are even more reluctant to approach – forgiving ourselves. We choose to not even see this by focusing on the other person's illness, but the inner twist is that all of this is tied up with how much we value our own being. Many people have inner fears that they have failed to draw the love of others, especially of their parents – which is usually where our foundations of love first falter. If we were not loved enough, or even at all, when we were young, then we are in grave danger of being unforgiving of ourselves.

It is all part of that human defense mechanism which conveniently passes the blame to others for what we don't like or fear in ourselves. Being unlovable, in our own eyes, can be a lifelong sentence unless we bring in the light of understanding and see how our parents were lost in their own wounds. That is what therapy is all about – seeing and releasing others from their failings and consequently releasing ourselves from blame. If parents fail to love sufficiently, their children carry those wounds. Children are not unloved or insufficiently loved because they failed to be the right child. They simply failed to have the right parent. As simple as that is, it is very hard for those adult children to forgive themselves for having an insufficient parent. With proper guidance, those adult children can grow to understand that their parents did what they were trained to do.

Even today, many people refuse to look at these issues. If a caregiver is someone who has not found understanding and forgiveness, then heaven help the person they look after. The danger is that they then become an insufficient parent to the parent who needs care. What happens is the result of what happened to their own parents – the sins of the fathers being visited upon the children even unto the third and fourth generation.

The unwinding of this terrible rope begins when an adult grows up enough to risk looking at their own pain and finally admitting that they did not deserve what happened. They did not do wrong; they were not the wrong child. The root of all this healing is forgiveness, and that forgiveness must first of all be directed inwardly. Once we start on that road, we find so much to forgive – ourselves, our family, even our family members who show pitiable weakness by falling prey to demeaning illnesses like dementia. An illness which basically says, can you love me as I am?

It hurts to watch people once competent and admired become more unkempt, much less able, fading reflections of themselves. Sitting with sorrow isn't something we do very much in our society, certainly not willingly. So how can we temper our sorrow and put aside our blaming? There is only one way I know of – sit with it by sitting with the person who has dementia.

Coming Into the Here and Now

- Sit quietly in the here and now
- Let go of the past in this moment
- Let go of pictures of the future, which is completely unknown to you
- Breathe gently, slowly, in and out
- What feeling you have, let it be your feeling
- When you're ready to speak truth, speak

We are afraid of speaking the truth to a person with Alzheimer's. We think we'll hurt this person by talking about it, but that is all part of our deep confusion about this illness. It is having Alzheimer's that hurts, not talking about having it.

And it hurts more when people avoid truth and avoid us as we are now. If you've avoided this kind of conversation, you might be pleasantly surprised at the conversations you can have with a person with dementia.

You can deal with your own fear of dementia by making friends with this person here and now. Be willing to sit with them. Be willing to sit with your own feelings and listen to the pain inside your own heart. Everything your elder has ever been, he or she still is. It is not accessible, in the reliable old ways, but the heart, the spirit, and the deep essential being still lives within.

In fact, so many of our ways of seeing them as failed people have much more to do with who we are, not who they are. They aren't less loving; in fact they are often more. The heart can become very open and warm and feeling in a person with dementia. Medical jargon calls it labile, but I call it feeling their feelings.

We think of them as useless, but how useful are you during your average day? What did you do for world peace today? In fact, were you yourself peaceful at all today? What is it that you want from this person with dementia? Maybe you just wanted life to go on as always, so you didn't have to pay attention to your mother or your grandmother. Maybe some of this anger that people feel is just that there is now one more thing to be added to the daily load of being human.

Perhaps if you learned how to visit a person with dementia, that might help you deal with your inner feelings. Here are my suggestions for you to find that real person inside.

How to Visit Someone with Alzheimer's

Leave your pity at home and take your heart with you. No matter how poor a person's memory, the heart is always within. Always. Your task will be to engage that heart.

Begin by slowing down, and then introduce yourself. No matter if this is your grandma who you've known forever.

"Hi, Grandma, this is your granddaughter Tiffany. How are you?" is a perfect introduction for a person with Alzheimer's. No memory questions, please. Your grandmother doesn't forget your name to tease you, nor to secretly tell you she doesn't love you any more. Her brain function cannot support her memory – that's all. Seek hints of her love by looking in her eyes, holding her hand, listening with your heart.

All too often I have heard family members say, "We don't visit Grandma anymore. She doesn't know us now."

My question to that is always, "But don't *you* know her? Don't you think she needs love until the day she dies?"

Who will give her that love if not her family? Yes, I know it's painful to see her no longer the woman she was, but get over yourself. A lot of life is painful. Grow up. Nothing is as painful as being abandoned by family and friends just when you need them most.

Having Alzheimer's is curiously contagious, apparently – it gives everyone else memory problems. As someone who has lived and worked with people with Alzheimer's for nearly two decades, I have to tell you I am tired of hearing that Alzheimer's is mainly a disease that is painful for families.

It is most painful of all for the person with dementia. Why not concentrate on bringing that person love and warmth and entertainment, and creating a special moment in the loneliness that is Alzheimer's? When you visit people with dementia, bring food, photos, and a project to share, and be prepared to take things slowly.

Look them in the eye, slow down a lot, and touch them often. Project warmth and a loving heart. Compliment them. Talk about things they know. Come into the present moment with them, even if their present moment is 1926. If you take photos, take old photos of their own parents and siblings. Your children's pictures may not mean so much.

People with Alzheimer's live in the past a lot. That is their appropriate home, where they do their work of memory. Walk with them in that place. This world and your life may mean very little to them. Accept what they tell you and nod and look interested.

When they tell you the alligators are in the creek today, and they live in Sierra Vista, Arizona, just say, "Really?" Don't correct them – which they will ignore anyway. You don't have to agree with them either. Just be interested.

"Really – buffalo? Over the hill this morning, you say? My goodness!"

If they tell you dead relatives came to visit, just be interested. Dead relatives often visit the very old as they near their death. It's not craziness. Don't keep correcting people with dementia. They have dementia, for goodness sake. Just be accepting and bring your sense of humor – laughter improves the functioning level of brains with dementia. You will not in any degree make people worse by *not* correcting them. Neither will you improve their functioning by correcting them. In fact, you will make them nervous.

Making them better is not your job. Just be with them as they are. If they say wondrous things, why, just enjoy it. Don't hold onto who they used to be. Just find the treasure in them now. Entertain them. I used to read tabloids to the old ladies in my Alzheimer's care home in Portland – the ones in which Big Foot married a Martian and a new set of Ten Commandments had been found under Mount Shasta.

They loved the stories. They loved poems with a good rhythm and those *Reader's Digest* snippets. Try those if you don't know how to start a conversation. Bring cookies. Bring ice-cream treats. Give a hand massage or a shoulder-rub. Be a wonderful gift to them. Tell them things you enjoy about them. These are people who have lost their value to almost everyone in the world. Show them what you value about them.

One day, you too will be older, less able. Do you want to be judged as less valuable and less lovable because of your shortcomings? Shortcomings, moreover, not of character or morals, but just the stuff of age. We are so merciless to the old.

How about practicing loving-kindness with that person you know? Your family will be watching and this is how you teach them to value people simply because you love them. Chances are, if you do that, they'll still remember you when you can't even get their names right.

People with Alzheimer's want to be loved, secure, and appreciated. Just like the rest of us. In fact, it is what we have in common with them that we hate and fear. We are angered by their neediness, their loneliness, their being so dependent on uncertain people like ourselves. We don't love them and we feel deeply that this is what it is like to be so lost and dependent. If we have any roots in such deep and unwelcome feelings, then a person with dementia pushes all our buttons.

If we have the courage to sit with them in their moments of being, we find healing for ourselves. Our own compassion answers our deep fear.

There will be loving understanding for us should we ever become this person. We become our own good example by doing the thing that is needed. We start, so that we shall be loved, even if there's nothing about us that seems to deserve it.

So, take yourself in hand and bring self-discipline to your own negative feelings. Choose not to be angry, root out your fear and look at its nature, live in its presence and see that it is only a feeling. It may ripple through us like a dark tide but it is not who we really are.

When we sit with someone with dementia and seek their own deep humanness, we also find our own. We are all great souls. We just have to choose to live that way.

Maybe it helps to realize how many of us there are. We are caregivers, all over the country, all over the continent, all over the world. We get up in the night to sit with someone who is distressed or in pain. We make a baby's meal for an old woman and feed it spoonful by spoonful. We feel overwhelmed. We are often poor. We are sometimes lonely in this work, but that is because we mistakenly think we are alone.

We are an army – an army of caregivers. We are all out here somewhere. Know it and feel it, friend. Every spiritual tradition in the world includes the sacred path of caregivers. Muslim, Christian, Jewish, Buddhist, Hindu – everyone recognizes the sacred journey of the caregiver. We grow in soul by walking this path.

We are all out here, so think about us all when you feel lonely or wonder what on earth you're doing or how you'll do it. Remember we are all out here, on a journey as a companion with the courage to go with someone to the gates of death. Send a loving thought or a prayer to us, as we send them to you.

We are all out here, in small towns and isolated cabins, in cities alight all night, by the oceans and in the mountains. We are everywhere. Choose to belong to us all, this great and growing army of caregivers – we who do the sacred work of caring, even in the face of death and even when we're tired. We all carry you in our hearts and we ask that you do the same. Not one of us is really ever alone once we realize how many of us there are.

A LIFE IN ALZHEIMER'S LAND

It takes a great soul to love and care for a parent with whom there are still unresolved issues of need and pain. Fortunately, there are great souls out there. I have met a lot of them since that time with Hannah.

As Hannah's life gradually unfolded for me, I came to understand why we were connected at the heart. We had profound issues in common, though they had very different dramas around them. I was only beginning to learn that when you are a caregiver to someone, you really get to know who they are at their deepest levels.

As an Alzheimer's caregiver, you see people stripped down to the depths of their hearts. Often you find out then just what it is that you have in common and out of that comes the deep love that we caregivers often feel for those we care for. We meet them at the banks of the River Lethe. We learn what it is they have to forget and we find out what they remember. Their hearts are stripped naked. That is why people fear Alzheimer's.

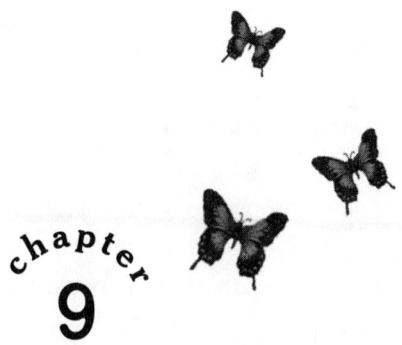

The Alzheimer Work
of the Soul

All human beings have great soul work to undertake in this span of human life. We have to do our work of loving. Should we live to old age, and these days most of us do, then we have to undertake the task of coming to understanding, peace, and reconciliation with the journey of our life. And we have to answer the great question: "How much did I love?"

If people know, understand, and nurture their spiritual journey, their lives are richer, deeper, and warmer. Whatever happens, love is our defense against the difficulties of life itself. That is true for most human beings, but is it true for people with Alzheimer's? After all, they cannot remember, they cannot be rational, they cannot work things out for themselves, and they are living in a state of helplessness. Or are they?

Hannah was the first person with Alzheimer's I ever looked after. She was a German-Jewish refugee in Berkeley, California, seventy-nine years old, diagnosed with Alzheimer's at the age of seventy-four.

I was fascinated by Hannah's dilemma. She had no reliable access to her own memories. It meant not only that her own life history was fractured, but also that she had lost the means to organize her own present. Knowing to bathe, to dress, how to cook, simply knowing what comes next or what happened yesterday – it was all gone. One day, she was really struggling painfully to remember something.

"I'm so sorry, Hannah," I said, "It must be so hard not to be able to get out what it is in your mind."

She nodded. "Yes," she said. "It is hard. It is. But I have many things also in my heart."

That was certainly true and because she was the first person I had ever known with Alzheimer's, that was a great teaching. There were other interesting things I learned from Hannah, too. She did not know and could not remember the names of any of us who looked after her. At first, I felt a little sad about this and then I noticed something. She would come close to me, peer into my face, and then a light of recognition dawned.

"Ah!" she cried delightedly, "It's you! I'm so glad!"

This was how it became clear to me that there were different kinds of memory. The biodata memory was pretty much destroyed. The sense-of-the-familiar memory was available with variable access. Then I also noticed that when I helped her get dressed – without which she might put her socks on her hands – she found it hard at first. Then suddenly she slipped into an old, well-established body habit that led her successfully through the rest of the process. Clearly there was also a sense memory that could be accessed. To access these different kinds of memory, Hannah needed time and no stress.

She enjoyed routine. It had its own sense of security that outlasted memory. She did not remember what she did yesterday, but doing it again today soothed her. Routine supplied a structure that her memory could not, as if her heart and body could taste comfort in the repetitions of life. That was how I learned that people with dementia have access to more ways of knowing than most of us realize. How something feels is also a reliable source of internal information for them.

After Hannah's family decided to put her into long-term care, I went on to work in a large Alzheimer's facility in Alameda. Over fifty residents lived there. I began to realize how many of them had lived dramatically traumatized lives. This was when I began to ask myself whether their dementia was in some way a response to the stress of those difficult lives.

There was Melia, who had passed her entire childhood in a concentration camp where seven of her nine siblings died, as did her mother and her father. She was four when her father was picked out of the men's line to be sent into the gas chamber for execution.

"Look after your little sister," he said to his children before calmly walking to his fate.

Melia would sit in her wheelchair and shout, "Help! Help!" When anyone went over to find out what she needed, she just smiled and shook her head, looking very cheerful. This behaviour would irritate the staff, but I felt I could perhaps understand why a woman with her terrible childhood could just have a need to yell "Help!" and have people come to her aid, over and over again. I could see how this was a deep resolution of terrible trauma.

There was Nellie, raped and made pregnant by a farmhand on her parents' farm when she was just thirteen years old. She was then sent away in disgrace by her fundamentalist Christian family for being a bad girl, to have her illegitimate baby. Sometimes on her bad days I would hear her calling out, "I'm not a wicked girl. I'm not!"

Then there was Mildred, a tiny, cheerful eighty-seven-year-old who spent much of her time cleaning the nursing home, dusting and wiping surfaces as she had done during her long life as a homemaker. Once, as I was walking past a closet, a thin bony hand reached out from inside and grabbed my wrist.

"Oh my gosh!" I gasped. "Mildred, you'll give me a heart attack!"

"Is my daddy out there?" she whispered.

"No, no, he's not," I stammered.

"He's trying to hurt me," she was still whispering. "I know he hurt my mamma. I saw the bruises on her face. Is he there?"

"No, Mildred, your daddy isn't here to hurt you any more," I said more firmly now, as I put my arm about her shoulders. "You're safe here. No one's going to hurt you."

But that wasn't entirely true. It couldn't be, because her own memories hurt her. They were the memories she had to keep living with until their power to hurt her was gone. She taught me that these old, frail, haunted children have to speak their truth until the story has lost its power to wound them. Maybe until they die.

Sometimes people achieve that kind of resolution. Sometimes the very care and tenderness they receive during the closing years of their lives heals those wounds. Sometimes the love of their caregivers is what heals them. I began to see that this was not just a stray memory circuit, aimlessly weaving the same life moment through consciousness.

This was how the mind of a person with dementia did its best to seek and bring about healing. People with reliable memories, who know the difference between life and time, can choose to see therapists. Old people with dementia, however, do not lose their chance to heal as well, although they may well do splendidly with a talk therapist, too.

Actually, the more I have observed people working with these issues of trauma, I have sometimes wondered whether dementia was a refuge in which they found a freedom to do nothing but seek their healing. Unable to continue everyday life as they had known it, they were now free to wander in the areas of life where their attention was truly needed. Human beings are essentially designed for being well and healing from illness and accident. We aren't like flowers that lose their petals in a storm. We can and do survive a great deal and can still come to a healing deep enough to allow us to get on with some kind of life.

We have strong souls. Perhaps our resilient nature struggles even in the midst of dementia to push us towards healing. Talk therapy is all about having a witness to the human story. Being heard brings its own kind of healing. The oft-repeated trauma stories of people with dementia surely are seeking much the same from those who listen to them. I remember Sarah as I write this, a woman who attended the Alzheimer day-care project I set up in Florence, Oregon.

It was just a small program, with never more than ten people a day, but I managed to get some federal funding in 1993 via the Robert Wood Johnson Foundation (RWJF) Partners in Caregiving grant for the Dementia Services Program national program. Sarah was a cheerful woman who enjoyed coming. We sat around one long table and got on with all the various activity projects designed to amuse and involve people while they socialized with each other.

A person with dementia can really be comforted by the company of others just like them. It lowers the general stress level of their lives. On one particular day Sarah seemed preoccupied. She didn't work on the big collage we were putting together, but kept picking at a roll of toilet paper on the table that we used for wiping up paint.

Pick, pick, she went. Pick, pick, pulling tiny little fragments of paper off the roll. I was feeling a bit irritated with her for demolishing the roll in that way. Pick, pick.

"When I was young," she started hesitantly, picking away, "There was ... we ... I."

She stopped. Pick, pick. I wanted to snatch that poor toilet roll away from her. Why was she doing this?

"We went ... it was one Sunday. We went ... it was a picnic. A church picnic."

Everyone stopped and looked at Sarah as she stripped some more paper off the toilet roll.

"Well, I had ... I wanted to ... it was ..." Pick, pick.

She was thirteen, a girl at the Baptist Church picnic – in the woods. She needed to go to the toilet but she did not know these woods. The kindly Baptist minister took her to find the toilets, took her inside the toilet, and sexually assaulted her.

"If you say anything about this," he said sternly, "God will send you straight to Hell for being a bad girl." He told her to clean herself up and stop crying.

Once she finished telling us this story in fits and starts, Sarah covered her eyes and wept helplessly, like a small child. She had never, ever told anyone this story of what had happened to her. Everyone comforted her. I thought to myself, no wonder it was toilet paper that triggered her to tell us this. We all assured her that, no, she would not go to Hell for telling us now.

"You did nothing wrong," I said. "He was the one who was wrong. He might have been a Baptist minister but he was a bad man and what he did was bad. You weren't bad. It wasn't you."

It was extraordinary how much better Sarah seemed in the weeks that followed. She had laid a terrible burden of secrecy and shame aside and finally came to feel that perhaps she would not go to Hell for being molested after all.

As a caregiver, you never know when you might be entrusted with the hidden stories that burden a person's heart. When it happens, our task is not to try to make it right, but to validate and support this person, to allow the anger or grief that goes with hard truths and deep secrets. We must honor the weight of the secret they share with us and respect their courage.

Only after that do we offer comfort. The most important thing for a caregiver to know is that such work is very healing. Allowing people to tell upsetting things is not upsetting for them. It comforts them. Even if they weep, they are still comforted because their tears are tears that lead to peace within.

"My dad keeps telling us how he watched his little brother drown when he was seven. How often do we have to listen to this?" asks Steve.

A person with dementia tells the story of a trauma as many times as he needs for the story to be told. Only when it loses its pain is that story over. For some people, this might be a finite number of times, after which it is a settled issue. Or the story might have to be told several times every day for the rest of this person's life.

Perhaps caregivers would accept this repetition more easily if they realized there really is purpose in the process. It serves the same purpose as flashbacks. In fact, it is a kind of flashback, calling this person's attention to a trauma that has not yet been healed.

This is not the only way in which people with dementia seek healing for themselves. In part, it is their disease that pushes them towards other healing paths. Losing the strictly rational from life can often free a person to live a more heart-centered life. People with dementia commonly become much more open with their emotions and are often more loving than they've ever been before.

Skills and abilities may be drastically curtailed, but emotional availability increases. With this openness often comes great sensitivity. Dementia often makes people profoundly alert to people's feelings, and they have unwavering radar for the emotions of others. Many caregivers have experienced coming to work in a bad mood but thought they were disguising it from the person they cared for. Then that person threw an anger tantrum as if to confront them with themselves.

Often caregivers report that the people they care for seem almost psychic at times, honing right in on a particular issue which has never been discussed but which preoccupies the caregiver.

Another observation I made was that often people seemed to have dementia to a degree of impairment that matched the degree of emotional need within this person. For example, all the people I have known who became bed-ridden and largely unable to self-care at all were almost invariably born into severely difficult family circumstances. Little or no nurturing care was given to them as a newborn. Adult life was problem-ridden.

When we care for an elder who needs to be looked after like an infant, we bring healing to that deep woundedness. Our care has spiritual and emotional meaning. We are giving something that was never before experienced by this person – unconditional love. It is very important for family caregivers to understand this. It brings them great comfort when they understand their care is a profoundly meaningful gift to this person.

Great Alzheimer's Themes

When people have dementia, we often see them involved with some of the great themes of human life and this is not accidental. Everyone thinks about these things, especially as they age. If you ask competent elders over eighty, they'll tell you they think about these issues a great deal in the privacy of their own minds and hearts. Those who have dementia just process that thinking in more visible and sometimes uncontrolled ways, consistent with their illness. An old woman with dementia might weep like a child because she longs for her mother to hold her. An elder without dementia might have dreams in which she meets her mother and talks with her.

Home: This is not only one of the great themes in everybody's life, but it is also one of the most annoying for the caregivers of people with dementia. Many people's sun-downing themes involve some aspect of home – wanting to go home, feeling that people are expecting them at home, wondering where home is.

Sometimes caregivers assume that home is the last address this person lived at and that's where everyone is waiting, but that is probably not so. Once people move into deep Alzheimer's, they also move into limitless, timeless territory, and this means entering the archetype of home.

Home as a great Alzheimer's theme usually represents security, safety, nurturing, and love, so the person will choose the place that represents those longings. Usually it is the parental home, North Dakota prairie, 1931. Sometimes it will be the home this person shared with a young spouse, where the new baby lay sleeping.

The longing is to experience what I call "homeness," a feeling that safety and love enfold us. Remember, having dementia means never feeling at home again, even in your own life. No reliable memory to keep your story around you, no loving, familiar family members to protect you, no sense of what it is you do in daily life. People get totally lost even in their own lives and, should they go to a care facility, they experience being one hundred times more lost.

There comes a time when the word "home" comes to represent preparing for or longing to meet death, to go home to God, to move on to where everyone else in the family went. Whether or not this person actually had any specific religious or spiritual beliefs, that same expression "home" will still be used.

Understanding the concept in its largest, almost mythic sense helps caregivers deal better with the demand, insistence, or oft-repeated yearning to be or go home. Instead of arguing about it, which will get you nowhere and only upset the person you look after, validate the feeling without getting into a factual struggle.

"I want to go home."

"I'm sorry. You must really be missing your family now."

Caregivers are often afraid to do this, but it is usually notably successful. Even if the person starts to weep, don't worry. Weeping is appropriate for loneliness, fear, and a sense of loss. Let the tears come, be empathetic, give time and some Kleenex, and you might be surprised how much better this person feels afterwards. People might be demented, but the feelings are real and we need to help them on the level of feeling, not on the more superficial level of their dementia.

What people are really saying when they talk about home is that they don't belong anywhere anymore. And that is true, so our comfort needs to come at that level. Don't tell them this care facility is their home now. Don't tell them anything factual. Be empathetic. Be like a mother to them.

Realize that they are suffering and feel just like a lost and unmothered child. That feeling is authentic.

Belonging: This is a cause of a great deal of the emotional distress in dementia. Our memory supplies so much of our sense of belonging in life. Without reliable memory, it is easy for people to feel they don't belong anywhere.

It is also a question in anyone's life – where do we belong, who do we belong with, how do we find out how to belong? It all gets ripped away in dementia. Loneliness and a sense of being adrift can easily overtake people. You've seen them – people sitting lonely right there in the middle of their own family, with nothing to do and nowhere that they can remember to go.

There's a lot we can do and much of it is obvious and simple. Give this person your time and concentrated attention on a regular basis. Give this person something to do, even if they'll do it badly. So what? Everyone needs some way to make a contribution.

Belonging is not just a social feeling or a place to be. It is also having helpful and meaningful things to do. It is being of value and being valued, a sense of well-being, which we caregivers can enhance if we take the trouble to reach out and ask folks to help us. Some won't, but those who will feel so glad to be needed.

Parents: Even orphans think about parents. Even people who have bad parents think about good parents. Having a mother and a father is essential for the deep well-being of children, even at the spiritual level.

Did you know that the ancient Hebrew word for God has linguistic roots for male and female in it and therefore, ideally and scholastically, should be translated as Father-Mother-God? This tells you how deep in humans is the longing for a mother and a father. Old people with dementia, often in difficult and lonely circumstances, of course long for their parents. Someone has to be their mother and their father, and perhaps especially their mother. Talk of parents, therefore, is usually a sign of this person's emotional need.

Therefore, when your elder asks where his mother is, don't tell him "dead." Instead, be vague and evasive and act motherly. If you're a guy, acting motherly means moving in, making comforting physical contact, and being soothing. That's what mothers do for infants in distress.

A little of this goes a long way. After a short while, you can re-direct the energy to eating, moving, or maybe a ride in the car, and this will do the trick. The blessing of dementia is the same as its curse – short-term memory. This means you can easily use bribery, persuasion, or re-direction to recapture this person's energy because they will probably have forgotten their distress in about ten minutes.

We've already looked at the necessity of dealing with trauma, but the converse is that it can also be very healing to re-live our memories of good times, enjoyable events, and great personal achievements. The audience participation requires support, interest, and recognition, however many times you've already heard it.

This resolution process is not all pain. I think of Orelia, with whom I walked for her ninetieth year. If I had listened to what everyone else said, including the relatives who loved her, I might have thought that she, with her dementia, was empty and doing nothing. If I had listened to those who knew her before, I might have viewed this time in her life as confused, demeaning, and dysfunctional, as they did. Instead, I saw her heart and concentration fully involved with her inner work. The rest is just the stuff we need to forgive of the very old – their incapacities – just as I hope they forgive our shallow judgments about their lives.

Many a person manages to live in old age with limitations that would have seemed unbearable even to themselves at an earlier time. Our souls are great and they expand their tolerance for difficulty when life demands it.

Now it takes Orelia an hour to get up and an hour to make her bed, but she has those hours available, so it doesn't seem a hardship. If Orelia is haunted by anything, she does not reveal it. Instead, she weaves together the lines of her times, often quite seamlessly. She shows some of the nonsense we talk of when we talk of Alzheimer's.

Oh yes, we say, she has delusions. This old woman brings together stories of her past from very different times and places. But, after all, isn't it within her that all these elements meet? Her life itself is the time line and her memory is the frame of everything that comes together.

She ends her day with the ten o'clock news from Tucson. It starts with a story about illegal immigrants.

"Oh yes," she says. "They come from Europe, you know, and they're always trying to get in down the St. Lawrence River. Half the families in town employ them. Well, they work hard, you know."

Of course, she is referring to 1925, Rochester, New York, up near the Canadian border, the town where she was born, not to 2005, Sierra Vista, near the Mexican border. The next item is about the police catching drunk drivers over the holiday weekend.

"Ah," she says wisely, "it's because of Prohibition. They go out and get drunk in the speakeasies." I smile to myself as I think of the speakeasies of Sierra Vista. Then, just as I'm getting used to the time and the setting – Rochester, 1920s – on comes Elton John.

"That's Elton John – my, he got fat!" Orelia says, throwing me completely back into the present. "Do you know 'Fatty' Arbuckle?" she spins me back.

"No, but I've heard of him," I offer.

"I haven't seen him lately," she muses. "I wonder if he's still making films. I don't think they make comedies anymore, do they?"

"Well, er ..." I start.

"They don't make musicals now either. I suppose they stopped writing songs," she continues, but it seems to be a philosophical observation, not a complaint. I let it pass. I have a vast repertoire of non-committal comments for these times, the politer-sounding British version of "Yeah, right!"

"Oh really? You don't say? Is that right? My goodness! Well, I never! That's interesting."

I try to learn my own old-age lessons in advance from those I work with. If I apply Orelia's lessons, they would be something like this: keep smiling, don't complain, sing cheerful songs, stick to your schedule, keep a pet, be nice to the young in your family so they'll love you when you get old, cultivate the power of denial, do what you like, ignore what you don't, keep up with the news, drink plenty of orange juice, and eat Oreos in the middle of the night.

Bliss: Bliss is not something you need to talk about, but when you see it on the face or in the eyes of someone you care for, be happy with and for them.

This is what many people come to after journeying through the pain, fear, anger, and losses of this illness. They may come to peace, joy, and, yes, even a sense of bliss. You have every reason to be hopeful it can come to someone you care about. With enough support from us, enough acceptance of the struggles of this person's life, enough kindness, we can sometimes walk with them towards this great spiritual happiness.

This is when the person arrives at a sense of being enfolded in unconditional love. As a caregiver, you need never lose hope that peace and a full heart will come to this person you care for. It doesn't all depend on us, but we certainly can help the process, and in doing so, we can help ourselves. A great deal of the caregiver's path is about being in your own heart while others do their journey. It is difficult to find that still place inside sometimes, and sometimes it's hard all of the time.

We can't live so close to other people's pain and losses and fear without being deeply touched in all those areas ourselves. Besides which, the great majority of people who choose to be caregivers are deeply drawn to the task of helping others in their dark times of struggle.

Even for family caregivers, this is true. The one who is the family caregiver is usually self-appointed. Often this has been the one who was the good child, the one who tried to make Mom feel better, the one who watched and waited through fear and childhood loss while family life flowed in turmoil around them.

Adult caregivers were usually the childhood caregivers, too, and this is no coincidence. They are the ones who are drawn to making peace, to finding healing, and frankly, usually no one needs it more than they do. In families, there are usually those who do the caregiving and those who don't, and this can seem so very unfair. Others seem to get off free, without putting in effort, money, or even a brief appearance. However, it is those who turn up to do the job that get the chance at the great prize.

The prize is that they grow their heart and soul.

A LIFE IN ALZHEIMER'S LAND

If only everyone had the courage to really get to know who people are at the edge of the river. If only we saw the courage, the depth of being, and the determination of that human being making life as meaningful as possible in spite of the limitations of the disease process. If only we could all think like Pooh Bear, as in this passage from The House at Pooh Corner:

"Rabbit's clever," said Pooh thoughtfully.

"Yes," said Piglet, "Rabbit's clever."

"And he has Brain."

"Yes," said Piglet, "Rabbit has Brain."

There was a long silence.

"I suppose," said Pooh, "that's why he never understands anything."

So the moral of this story is that it is much better to be a Pooh than a Rabbit and bring deep heartfelt understanding to our life as caregivers rather than rack our brains.

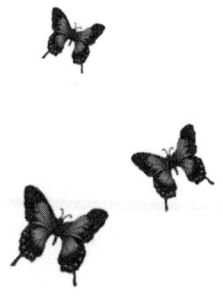

Epilogue

"Would you do me a favor?" asked the Activity Director, stopping me in the corridor one morning.

"If I can," I nodded.

"The poetry teacher's sick today and she can't come in, so I wonder if you'd do the poetry class in the Alzheimer's Unit."

"Me?" I said. "Well, I don't know a whole lot about writing poetry."

"Well, neither do most people here – and what they once knew they've probably forgotten, to be honest. I think the main thing is these days poetry's just what people make up as they go along. I mean, it doesn't have to rhyme or anything like that."

"Oh, that's a relief." I rolled my eyes. "Okay then, just as long as we don't have to make it rhyme."

She just laughed and went on her way.

"Now just how am I supposed to do a poetry class?" I muttered to myself.

Maria Black smiled at me. "Talking to yourself again? They say that's the first sign, don't they?"

Maria Black was a fine, dignified black woman with a big heart full of love and caring, even for the most ornery people in the Alzheimer's unit. She had worked there for fifteen years, from before it was even called the

Alzheimer's unit. She always did her best to bring love to the lonely souls in there.

"You know what, Maria? The Activity Director wants me to do the poetry class today. Do you know how they usually do it?" I knew we were probably not going to write a sonnet or even haiku.

"Well, I've seen that teacher with them and she usually takes something in with her – you know, like things from a kitchen or sometimes photographs – and she gets folks talking and then she writes down everything they say."

"And that's poetry?"

"Well, that's poetry in here anyway."

So I decided to round up some candidates for the class. I knew it had to be those who were likely to speak and not anyone who needed to keep walking for peace of mind. I guessed that I might find about nine people in the fifty-bed Alzheimer's unit who might be inveigled into coming to a poetry class. So I started my hunt. My first captive was Phyllis.

"Phyllis," I said cheerfully. "How are you today?"

"Oh, it's so good to see you," she said in her beautifully modulated voice, so ladylike and refined that you might expect her to wear a large flowery hat and a silk dress. She was not wearing her false teeth and her cardigan was ragged at the edges. It was painful to see her so neglected. I knew I would have to find out who her personal aide was so that we could track down her teeth. Then I would have to contact her public guardian to see if we could buy some clothes for her. She had a son but he had gone away to Alaska and seldom came. It would be easy to assume he did not care but undoubtedly it was not as simple as that. It can be very hard for the children of parents with Alzheimer's to find the courage to deal with what is going on.

The first time I met Phyllis she said, "My husband and I have just bought this hospital. My husband is a doctor and we have a beautiful apartment in the west wing."

"That's nice, Phyllis," I said, and I admired her for finding a way to dignify her life in this difficult time when she totally relied upon others to safeguard her well-being and her sense of self. Phyllis paints. Apparently she had never done anything like that before she came here. When her son brought her here, the staff thought she was going to die. It happens to about twenty-five percent of the people who come into long-term care. It is not their illness that they die of; I am sure about that. They die of transplant shock – the loss of everything familiar, just when they needed its support and framework for their unraveling lives. Their hearts fail them in these strange and disturbing surroundings.

"There is an inevitable attrition rate," the director of the facility said to me, which is just a way of saying it is not the fault of the facility.

I think it is the emotional chill that gets them, that and getting lost in the crowd. Being nothing in a big place when they once had a home they belonged in. Getting washed and dressed and being told to go here and get there. They die of the feeling that everything else has gone. They die of being lonely and feeling sad. They feel there is no more love for them and no more hope of love. They understand at a very deep level that there is nothing that can bring the change they want for themselves, that there is no point in hanging around.

That was how Phyllis looked when she arrived – as if she was going to die, sinking down inside and getting more pale and quiet until one morning Maria really thought for sure that Phyllis was going to die.

But that was the same day the art teacher came. He took hold of Phyllis's limp hand, stuck a paintbrush in it, and said, "Now, Phyllis, I want you to paint with this. I'm going to give you red paint and you're going to paint on this piece of paper."

And so she started painting. I have seen the paintings she did in her first three years. They might not be what a lot of people would think of as legitimate art. The art teacher brings outlines he has made of flowers or fish or houses or animals and he hands them out to people. Then he dips their brush in a color and puts the brush into their hand and points the end of the brush towards the paper and they do it from there. Their colors and their mixing and their lines go pell-mell onto the paper and come out looking totally different from each other.

Phyllis's work had a certainty and a richness of color about it that was beautiful. Her fish were radiant and demanding, her birds exotically daubed with brocaded patterns, her houses full and action-packed with blobs and stripes. Last year, she won the facility's painting competition and its fifty-dollar prize.

Recently her paintings have become pale and small and the lines have lost their confidence and life, and I wonder what that means. It worries me. I can see her slipping away. They do this before they die. Of course, they can die of anything, just like any old person. Even if they have Alzheimer's, they usually die of strokes and heart attacks and cancer and all the normal ailments of old age. But a lot of them go like Phyllis. They get quieter and quieter. They talk a whole lot less and they eat less and less and they sit still for long periods of time and eventually they stop. Just yesterday, I found Phyllis staring into the mirror in her room. She looked scared and lost.

"Who is that person?" she whispered to me.

"That's you, Phyllis," I whispered back, my arm around her poor thin shoulder. "That's you in the mirror."

"I'm nothing like that. I'm not old."

She sank down in her chair, as if I had told her bad news. Today, however, she seems restored and willing to come with me to the activity room. After I seat Phyllis safely at the table, I go out to the patio to fetch Louisa, who is sitting out there cursing at the sunshine.

"I don't care what you say," she rants, "I'll marry whoever I want to. I don't care. You can't stop me."

Since her medical record describes her as "a never-married woman," she must have lost that fight after all. I like Louisa. She is a feisty, rough-tongued old woman who apparently led a tough life. She was the only Caucasian woman working in small Chinese sweatshops in Oakland's China Town, earning her living as a seamstress. It is hard to imagine what depths of want led her into that situation, and she can no longer give a rational history of herself. It mainly comes in dramatic little outbursts from the soap opera of her life.

"Louisa, come on in and do some poetry," I said to her.

"Poetry? Poetry?" she roared at me. "You're so stupid – who the hell do you think you are? To hell with poetry!"

I felt a little bit the same way that morning, but I got her in place with some of the others anyway. I chose all the ones that could speak, even if they spoke in tiny high-pitched childish voices like Edna – who had never spoken that way until she developed dementia.

I still had no idea what I was going to do with them. However, as I was closing the patio door, I got my idea. There was one poor little Liquidamber tree out there, representing autumn all by itself. Its beautiful, big, five-fingered leaves were all turning scarlet and gold and a whole bunch of them had already collected at the bottom of its trunk.

I thought of it because there are no seasons inside the Alzheimer's care unit. No spring and no winter, no snow and no rain. Every day is the same as every other day. There are only lights on and lights off – those are the seasons. So it seemed an inspiration to bring a pile of those autumnal leaves inside.

They were sitting round the table in a slightly chaotic Alzheimer's way and I swept a bunch of those scarlet and gold leaves into my arms and dumped then down on the table. Then I swirled them all around so everyone had some leaves near them.

"Dirty slut!" said Louisa, with grim satisfaction. "You made the table all dirty – you're gonna get what for."

The rest of them loved those leaves. It was shocking for all of us to see them there. They made everything else in there look dead, they were so bright and sharp and scarlet and gold.

"Do you know what these are?" I asked.

Yes, they all knew. Leaves, leaves, they said, running their withered old hands through the wrinkly leaves.

"Do you know where they come from?"

They knew – trees, trees, they said – and you could see their thoughts going off into different directions as they touched them.

"Yes, trees," I said. "Do you like trees?"

"I like trees," Annie said. "Doesn't everyone?"

I wrote down what they were saying now.

"Why? Why do you like them?"

Esme said, "They do an awful lot for us."

"You should try them," Annie told me.

"Really? How should I try them?" I asked her.

"Lie under them and cool off." Esme poked me as she said that.

"I climbed up them when I was young," Annie mused. "I did. They were fruit trees. They were peaches, pears, apricots, cherries, and plums. We had a yard full of trees."

Molly grabbed a handful of leaves and she had a relaxed, gentle look on her face, unlike her usual dark, gloomy expression.

"What about you, Molly?" I asked. "You have a favorite tree?"

"Poplars are my favorite tree," she told me. "It was the green leaves. We had two in our front yard."

"Elms," said Annie. "The coloring in the leaves. You'd see autumn in the trees."

I took Molly's hand and I swirled it round over the leaves, all crackly.

"It was wonderful to be under the shade of a tree, lying there," she said so thoughtfully and peacefully that it touched my heart. "There were always birds. There were squirrels."

They all became a little quiet then, as if they had gone completely away from there to somewhere kind and serene.

I suddenly thought about the children's book I liked so much – *Where the Wild Things Are*. I liked the bit where the forest grew at night in the little boy Max's bedroom.

"What would you do if a forest grew in your room at night?"

"Stupid!" said Louisa. "You're stupid. You're crazy, you are!"

"I'd like it," whispered Phyllis. "I'd climb them."

"I wouldn't like a forest in my room," Annie shook her head. She had a very practical Italian nature. "I want a bed. The trees would hit the ceiling."

"You'd see the stars and the moon," Molly told her.

"They used to have orchards years ago," Annie said. "When the leaves were yellow, we went to the mountains to see them."

"When it's autumn, you want to cry," Phyllis said very quietly.

"You want to cry?" I asked. "Why?"

Phyllis leaned close and whispered, hesitating between phrases. "Seeing all these in their beauty – all so beautiful – and for such a short time we have them." She pushed her hands deep into the pile of gold and scarlet leaves and spoke so softly. I looked at her and saw that she had gone far, far away. Suddenly I knew she was telling me it wouldn't be long for her now.

"Come on, it's nearly lunch-time!" said one of the aides, breaking in. "We've got to set up the tables for lunch."

I sat behind the nursing station and I wrote it all out, nearly everything we said, pretty much the way we said it.

I like trees – doesn't everyone?

They do an awful lot for us.

Try them.

How shall we try them?

Lie under them and cool off.

I climbed up them when I was young.

I did.

They were fruit trees.

They were peaches, pears, apricots, cherries, and plums.

We had a yard full of trees.

Poplars are my favorite trees.

It was the green leaves.

We had two in our yard.

Elms...the coloring in the leaves.

You'd see autumn in the trees.

It was wonderful to be

Under the shade of a tree,

Lying there.

There were always birds,

There were squirrels.

If a forest grew in my room at night,

I'd like it. I'd climb the trees.

I wouldn't like a forest in my room.

I want a bed.

The trees would hit the ceiling.

You'd see the stars and the moon.

They used to have orchards years ago.

When the leaves were yellow,

We went to the mountains to see them.

When it's autumn, you want to cry.

You want to cry?

Why?

Seeing all these in their beauty...

All so beautiful...

And for such a short time we have them.

Three weeks later, Phyllis died as quiet and ladylike as she had lived, just slipping away in her sleep. And I had a poem they had created from the voices of their souls and the yearnings of their hearts. Not one of them knew the day, date, time, and year, but they all knew what was precious to them.

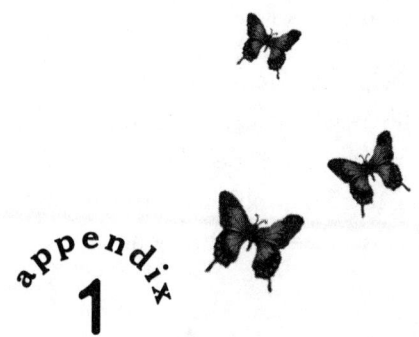

The Alzheimer's Work-Up

A complete Alzheimer's work-up is lengthy, sometimes taking more than one day to complete. Families should ask for a referral to a major Alzheimer's diagnostic center near where they live. No one can possibly diagnose Alzheimer's without such a work-up, because what we think of as Alzheimer's actually looks like a great many different conditions, from depression to hearing loss to liver trouble. The famous mini-mental test and clock-drawing test do not diagnose the presence of Alzheimer's, but just indicate that something significant is affecting memory and cognition.

Be sure you ask for the Age-Related Hydrocephalus test of fluid pressure on the brain. It is not always included unless you ask for it, though it should be. Increasingly researchers are finding that perhaps as many as twenty-five percent of everyone thought to have dementia actually has Age-Related Hydrocephalus, which can easily be treated with a low-risk minor procedure.

The workup includes very detailed information gathering, including:

- Questions about the person's general health, past medical problems, and ability to carry out daily activities

- Tests of memory, problem solving, attention, counting, and language

- Medical tests – such as tests of blood, urine, or spinal fluid
- Brain scans, including MRI and CAT scan

Sometimes, these test results help the doctor find other possible causes of the person's symptoms. This is why it is so important to have such a work-up. From fifteen to twenty percent of people have treatable, or even curable, conditions, such as thyroid problems, drug reactions, depression, brain tumors, and blood vessel disease in the brain.

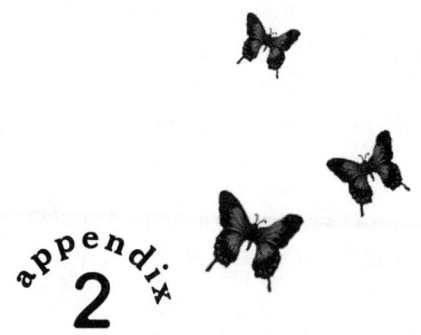

National Institute on Aging and Current Research

The National Institute on Aging (NIA) is part of the National Institute of Health (NIH) and serves as a central information resource on Alzheimer's disease. The NIA is the lead federal agency for AD research. This is how the NIH defines Alzheimer's on their website:

Dementia is a brain disorder that seriously affects a person's ability to carry out daily activities. The most common form of dementia among older people is Alzheimer's disease (AD), which initially involves the parts of the brain that control thought, memory, and language.

Scientists think that as many as 4.5 million Americans suffer from AD. The disease usually begins after age 60, and risk goes up with age.

While younger people also may get AD, it is much less common. About 5 percent of men and women ages 65 to 74 have AD, and nearly half of those age 85 and older may have the disease. It is important to note, however, that AD is not a normal part of aging.

AD is named after Dr. Alois Alzheimer, a German doctor. In 1906, Dr. Alzheimer noticed changes in the brain tissue of a woman who had died of an unusual mental illness. He found abnormal clumps (now called amyloid plaques) and tangled bundles of fibers (now called neurofibrillary tangles). Today, these plaques and tangles in the brain are considered signs of AD.

Scientists also have found other brain changes in people with AD. Nerve cells die in areas of the brain that are vital to memory and other mental abilities, and connections between nerve cells are disrupted. There also are lower levels of some of the chemicals in the brain that carry messages back and forth between nerve cells. AD may impair thinking and memory by disrupting these messages.

Alzheimer's is a slow disease process, and on average people live from eight to ten years after they are diagnosed. Some people may live for as many as twenty years.

While a definitive cure is not yet known, in the early and middle stages of the disease various medications may be able to help support brain and memory function. The usual drugs are donepezil (Aricept), rivastigmine (Exelon), or galantamine (Razadyne, previously known as Reminyl), but remember that new developments can come at any time. Currently, many approaches are aimed at replacing or enhancing deficient brain chemicals.

Some of the more difficult behaviors of Alzheimer's can be controlled with various other medications — for sleep, anxiety, and so on.

Drug Research

NIA-supported scientists are testing a number of drugs to see if they prevent or slow Alzheimer's disease, or can help reduce symptoms. Researchers undertake clinical trials to learn whether treatments that appear promising in observational and animal studies actually are safe and effective in people. Some ideas that seem promising turn out to have little or no benefit when they are carefully studied in a clinical trial.

Neuroimaging

Scientists are finding that damage to parts of the brain involved in memory, such as the hippocampus, can sometimes be seen on brain scans before symptoms of the disease occur. An NIA public-private partnership – the AD Neuroimaging Initiative (ADNI) – is a large study that will determine whether magnetic resonance imaging (MRI) and positron emission tomography (PET) scans, or other imaging or biological markers, can see early AD changes or measure disease progression. The project is designed to help speed clinical trials and find new ways to determine the effectiveness of treatments.

For more information on ADNI, call the NIA's Alzheimer's Disease Education and Referral Center at 1-800-438-4380, or visit www.alzheimers.nia.nih.gov.

Genetics

NIA is sponsoring the AD Genetics Study to learn more about risk factor genes for late-onset AD. To participate in this study, families with two or more living siblings diagnosed with AD should contact the National Cell Repository for AD toll-free at 1-800-526-2839. Information may also be requested through the study's website: http://ncrad.iu.edu.

Mild Cognitive Impairment

More recently, NIA scientists have focused on a type of memory change called mild cognitive impairment (MCI), which is different from both AD and normal age-related memory change.

People with MCI have ongoing memory problems, but they do not have other losses such as confusion, attention problems, and difficulty with language. The NIA-funded Memory Impairment Study compared donepezil, vitamin E, and placebo in participants with MCI to see whether drugs might delay or prevent progression to AD.

The study found that the group with MCI taking donepezil was at reduced risk of progressing to AD for the first eighteen months of a three-year study, when compared with their counterparts on placebo. However, the reduced risk disappeared after eighteen months, and by the end of the study, the probability of progressing to AD was the same in the two groups. Vitamin E had no effect at any time point in the study when compared with placebo.

Antioxidants

Additional studies are investigating whether antioxidants – vitamins E and C – can slow AD. Another clinical trial is examining whether

153

vitamin E and/or selenium supplements can prevent AD or cognitive decline.

Additional studies on other antioxidants are ongoing or being planned, including a study of antioxidant treatments – vitamins E and C, alpha-lipoic acid, and coenzyme Q – in patients with mild to moderate AD.

Gingko biloba

Early studies suggested that extracts from the leaves of the *Ginkgo biloba* tree may be of some help in treating AD symptoms. There is no evidence yet that *Ginkgo biloba* will cure or prevent AD, but scientists are now trying to find out in a clinical trial whether it can delay cognitive decline or prevent dementia in older people.

Clinical Trials

If you are interested in taking part in future clinical trials, contact the NIA. People with AD, those with MCI, or those with a family history of AD who want to help scientists test possible treatments may be able to take part in clinical trials. Healthy people also can help scientists learn more about the brain and AD. The NIA maintains the AD Clinical Trials Database, which lists AD clinical trials sponsored by various research bodies.

To find out more about these studies, contact the NIA's ADEAR Center at 1-800-438-4380 or visit the ADEAR Center website, www.nia.nih.gov/Alzheimers/ResearchInformation/ClinicalTrials. You also can sign up for email alerts on new clinical trials as they are added to the database. Additional clinical trials information is available at www.clinicaltrials.gov. You can keep tabs on NIH progress in the battle against Alzheimer's by telephone and on the Internet.

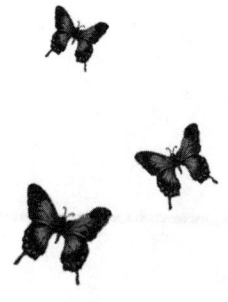

Resources

Organizations

I. The National Institute of Health (NIH) includes the National Institute on Aging (NIA), which serves as a central information resource on Alzheimer's disease. Their website – www.nia.nih.gov/alzheimers – has news and updates on Alzheimer's issues, including diagnosis, treatment, and care. You may also find advice on caregiving and long-term care. See Appendix II for more information on the NIA.

II. The primary resource for support of families and caregivers of those with Alzheimer's disease in the United States is the Alzheimer's Association. It has a national office and help-line as well as chapters in every state. It provides news and tips on its web site. The association also hosts support groups in many areas. Each state and regional office can put you into contact with local Alzheimer's Association chapters and support groups. There are almost three hundred local chapters that may assist people in finding the help they need.

Alzheimer's Association National Office

225 N. Michigan Ave., Fl. 17
Chicago, IL 60601
24/7 national toll-free help-line number: 1-800-272-3900

Illinois toll-free number: 1-800-621-0379
Website address: www.alz.org
Email address: info@alz.org

Alabama

117A Longwood Dr. SE
Huntsville, AL 35801
Phone: 256-880-1575

Arizona Desert Southwest Chapter – Arizona and Southern Nevada

1028 E. McDowell Rd.
Phoenix AZ 85006
Phone: 602-528-0545

California

1528 Chapala Street, Suite 204
Santa Barbara, CA 93101
Phone: 805-892-4259

5900 Wilshire Blvd., Suite 1100
Los Angeles, CA 90036
Phone: 323-938-3379

17771 Cowan, Suite 200
Irvine, CA 92614
Phone: 949-955-9000

4950 Murphy Canyon Road, Suite 250
San Diego, CA 92123
Phone: 858-492-4400

Colorado

455 Sherman Street, Suite 500
Denver, CO 80203
Phone: 303-813-1669

Connecticut
279 New Britain Road, Suite 5
Kensington, CT 06037
Phone: 860-828-2828

Florida
988 Woodcock Road, Suite 200
Orlando, FL 32803-3715
Phone: 407-228-4299

9365 U.S. Hwy. 19 N., Suite B
Pinellas Park, FL 33782
Phone: 727-578-2558

3333 Forest Hill Blvd., Suite 101
West Palm Beach, FL 33406
Phone: 800-861-7826

Georgia
1925 Century Boulevard, Suite 10
Atlanta, GA 30345
Phone: 404-728-1181

Great Plains
5601 South 27th Street, Suite 201
Lincoln, NE 68512
Phone: 402-420-2540

Hawaii
1050 Ala Moana Blvd., Suite 2610
Honolulu, HI 96814-4906
Phone: 808-591-2771

Idaho and Utah
855 East 4800 South, Suite 100
Salt Lake City, UT 84107
Phone: 801-265-1944

Illinois
606 West Glen Avenue
Peoria, IL 61614
Phone: 309-681-1100

8430 West Bryn Mawr, Suite 800
Chicago, IL 60631
Phone: 847-933-2413

Indiana
50 East 91st Street, Suite 100
Indianapolis, IN 46240
Phone: 317-575-9620

Iowa
1730 28th Street
West Des Moines, IA 50266
Phone: 515-440-2722

1570 42nd Street NE
Cedar Rapids, IA 52402
Phone: 319-294-9699

Kentucky
Kaden Tower,
6100 Dutchmans Lane, Suite 401
Louisville, KY 40205
Phone: 502-451-4266

Louisiana
3717 Government Street, Suite 7
Alexandria, LA 71302
Phone: 318-619-8383

Maine
170 U.S. Route 1, Suite 250
Falmouth, ME 04105
Phone: 207-772-0115

Massachusetts/New Hampshire
311 Arsenal Street
Watertown, MA 02472
Phone: 617-868-6718

Michigan
20300 Civic Center Drive, Suite 100
Southfield, MI 48076
Phone: 248-351-0280

310 North Main Street, Suite 100
Chelsea, MI 48118
Phone: 734-475-7043

Mid-South Chapter - North Alabama, NE, SE, Middle & West Tennessee
4205 Hillsboro Pike, Suite 216
Nashville, TN 37215-3439
Phone: 615-292-4938

Minnesota-North Dakota
4550 West 77th Street, Suite 200
Minneapolis, MN 55435
Phone: 952-830-0512

Mississippi

1900 Dunbarton Drive, Suite H
Jackson, MS 39216
Phone: 601-987-0020

Montana

3010 11th Avenue North
Billings, MT 59101
Phone: 406-252-3053

Nebraska and Iowa, Midlands

1941 South 42nd Street, Suite 205
Omaha, NE 68105
Phone: 402-502-4300

Nevada and Northern California

1060 La Avenida
Mountain View, CA 94043
Phone: 650-962-8111

New Mexico

9500 Montgomery NE, Suite 209
Albuquerque, NM 87111
Phone: 505-266-4473

New York

441 West Kirkpatrick Street
Syracuse, NY 13204-1361
Phone: 315-472-4201

2 Jefferson Plaza, Suite 103
Poughkeepsie, NY 12601
Phone: 800-872-0994

3281 Veterans Memorial Highway, Suite E-13
Ronkonkoma, NY 11779

Phone: 631-580-5100

360 Lexington Ave., 4th Floor
New York, NY 10017
Phone: 646-744-2900

85 Watervliet Avenue
Albany, NY 12206-2083
Phone: 518-438-2217

435 East Henrietta Road
Rochester, NY 14620
Phone: 585-760-5400

North Carolina
400 Oberlin Road, Suite 220
Raleigh, NC 27605
Phone: 919-832-3732 or 1-800-228-8738

3800 Shamrock Drive
Charlotte, NC 28215-3220
Phone: 704-532-7392

Ohio
3380 Tremont Road
Columbus, OH 43221
Phone: 614-457-6003

23215 Commerce Park Blvd., Suite 300
Beachwood, OH 44122
Phone: 216-721-8457

644 Linn Street, Suite 1026
Cincinnati, OH 45203
Phone: 513-721-4284

Oklahoma and Arkansas

6465 South Yale, Suite 312
Tulsa, OK 74136-7810
Phone: 918-481-7741

Oregon

1650 Northwest Naito Parkway, Suite 190
Portland, OR 97209
Phone: 503-416-0201

Pennsylvania

399 Market Street, Suite 102
Philadelphia, PA 19106
Phone: 215-561-2919

3544 North Progress Avenue, Suite 205
Harrisburg, PA 17110
Phone: 717-651-5020

Rhode Island

245 Waterman Street, Suite 306
Providence, RI 02906
Phone: 401-421-0008

Tennessee

326 Ellsworth
Memphis, TN 38111
Phone: 901-565-0011

201 W. Lincoln St.
Tullahoma, TN 37388
Phone: 931-455-3345

207 N. Boone Street, Suite 1500
Johnson City, TN 37604
Phone: 423-928-4080

7625 Hamilton Park Drive, Ste 8
Chattanooga, TN 37421
Phone: 423-265-3600

2200 Sutherland Ave.; Suite H102
Knoxville, TN 37919
Phone: 865-544-6288

4205 Hillsboro Pike, Suite 216
Nashville, TN 37215-3439
Phone: 615-292-4938

Texas
4144 N. Central Expressway, Suite 750
Dallas, TX 75204
Phone: 214-827-0062

2242 West Holcombe Blvd.
Houston, TX 77030-2008
Phone: 713-266-6400

101 Summit Avenue, Suite 300
Fort Worth, TX 76102
Phone: 817-336-4949

4687 North Mesa, Suite 200
El Paso, TX 79912
Phone: 915-544-1799

Vermont
172 North Main Street
Barre, VT 05641
Phone: 802-477-7000

Washington

910 West 5th Avenue, Suite 256
Spokane, WA 99204
Phone: 509-473-3390

12721 30th Avenue NE, Suite 101
Seattle, WA 98125-4312
Phone: 206-363-5500

Washington, D.C. Area

11240 Waples Mill Road, Suite 402
Fairfax, VA 22030
Phone: 703-359-4440

West Virginia

1111 Lee Street East
Charleston, WV 25301
Phone: 304-343-2717

Wisconsin

2900 Curry Lane, Suite A
Green Bay, WI 54311
Phone: 920-469-2110

517 North Segoe, Suite 301
Madison, WI 53705
Phone: 608-232-3400

6130 West National Avenue, Suite 200
Milwaukee, WI 53214
Phone: 414-479-8800

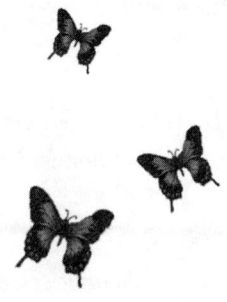

Books

The 36-Hour Day, 4th *edition: A Family Guide to Caring for People with Alzheimer Disease, Other Dementias, and Memory Loss in Later Life* by Nancy L. Mace and Peter V. Rabins. Baltimore, MD: Johns Hopkins University Press, 2006.

Alzheimer's: A Caregiver's Guide and Sourcebook by Howard Gruetzner. Hoboken, NJ: Wiley, 2001.

Alzheimer's & Dementia: Questions You Have…Answers You Need by Jennifer Hay. Allentown, PA: People's Medical Society, 1996.

Alzheimer's Disease: Frequently Asked Questions: Making Sense of the Journey by Frena Gray-Davidson. New York, NY: McGraw-Hill, 1999.

The Alzheimer's Sourcebook for Caregivers, 3rd edition: A Practical Guide for Getting Through the Day by Frena Gray-Davidson. New York, NY: McGraw-Hill, 1999.

Beating Alzheimer's: A Step Towards Unlocking the Mysteries of Brain Diseases by Tom Warren. Self-published paperback, still available online, 1991.

A Caregiver's Guide to Alzheimer's Disease: 300 Tips for Making Life Easier by Patricia R. Callone, ed. New York, NY: Demos Medical Publishing, 2005.

A Dignified Life: The Best Friends Approach to Alzheimer's Care, A Guide for Family Caregivers by Virginia Bell and David Troxel. Deerfield Beach, FL: HCI, 2002.

Learning to Speak Alzheimer's: A Groundbreaking Approach for Everyone Dealing with the Disease by Joanne Koenig Coste. Boston, MA: Mariner Books, Houghton Mifflin, 2004.

Travels in Place: A Journey into Memory Loss by Christiane W. Griffin-Wehr. Bandon, OR: Robert D. Reed Publishers, 2008.

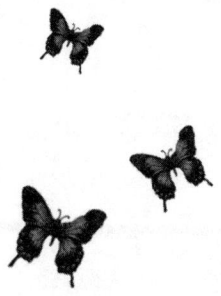

Websites

It is important to take advantage of all available resources so that you can offer the best care to your loved one. It can also ease the burden of caregiving. You can get advice from people who know what you're going through. They have experiences that you can learn from, and they can also point you to local services for help.

www.alzguide.com – author's website

www.healthcentral.com/alzheimers/websites

www.rideforalzheimers.com

www.thesavvyboomer.com/the_savvy_boomer/2008/01/alzheimers-care

www.alzheimers.about.com

www.alz.org/

www.alzheimers.org

www.ahaf.org/alzheimers

www.WellSpouse.org – a membership group that supports the wives, husbands, and partners of the ill or disabled

www.caregiving.com

www.caregiver.org – Family Caregiver Alliance (FCA): offers support for those who care for adults with Alzheimer's and other special needs.

www.alz.org

www.eldercare.gov – Eldercare Locator: This government resource helps older people and caregivers find the support services they need in their area.

www.caregiving.org

www.familycaregiverweb.com

www.caregivershome.com

www.care-givers.com

www.nhcoa.org – National Hispanic Council on Aging (NHCOA): The premier nonprofit organization in the nation, advocating on behalf of Hispanic older adults.

www.umm.edu/altmed/articles/dementia-000046.htm – University of Maryland Medical Center

www.abchomeopathy.com and www.hahnemannlabs.com – homeopathic remedies in the USA

www.helios.co.uk – homeopathic remedies in the UK

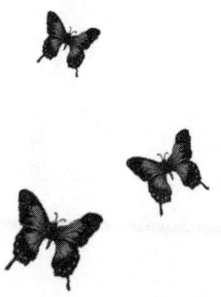

Area Agencies on Aging

Area Agencies on Aging were established by Congress under the Older Americans Act (OAA) in 1973 to respond to the needs of Americans sixty and over in every local community. AAAs provide services that help make it possible for older adults to remain in their homes and communities as long as possible. The following is a list of the AAAs by state, with the location of all local branches. Use your local telephone directory's state section for phone numbers and addresses of the nearest AAA.

Alabama
Alabama-Tombigbee AAA – Camden, AL
East Alabama Regional Planning and Development Com –
    Anniston, AL
Jefferson County Office of Senior Citizens – Birmingham, AL
Lee-Russell Council of Governments/AAA – Opelika, AL
North Central Alabama Regional Council of Governments –
    Decatur, AL
Northwest Alabama Council of Governments – Muscle Shoals, AL
South Alabama Regional Planning Commission – Mobile, AL
Southern Alabama Regional Council on Aging – Dothan, AL

TARCOG AAA – Huntsville, AL
West Alabama Regional Commission – Northport, AL

Alaska
Chugachmuit – Anchorage, AK
Maniilaq Association – Kotzebue, AK

Arizona
AAA Region One Inc. – Phoenix, AZ
Inter-Tribal Council of Arizona – Phoenix, AZ
NACOG-Area Agency on Aging – Flagstaff, AZ
Pima Council on Aging – Tucson, AZ
Pinal/Gila Council for Senior Citizens – Casa Grande, AZ
SEAGO AAA – Bisbee, AZ

Arkansas
AAA of Southeast Arkansas – Pine Bluff, AR
AAA of Southwest Arkansas Inc. – Magnolia, AR
AAA of Western Arkansas Inc. – Fort Smith, AR
Area Agency on Aging of Northwest Arkansas – Harrison, AR
Carelink Central Arkansas AAA Inc. – North Little Rock, AR
East Arkansas AAA Inc. – Jonesboro, AR
White River AAA – Batesville, AR

California
AAA Serving Napa-Solano – Vallejo, CA
Alameda County AAA – Oakland, CA
Area 12 AAA – Sonora, CA
Area 4 AAA – Sacramento, CA
Central Coast Commission for Senior Citizens – Santa Maria, CA
City of Los Angeles Dept. of Aging – Los Angeles, CA
Council on Aging Silicon Valley – San Jose, CA
Department of Aging and Community Services – Stockton, CA
El Dorado County AAA – Placerville, CA
Fresno-Madera AAA – Fresno, CA

Inyo Mono AAA – Bishop, CA
Los Angeles County AAA – Los Angeles, CA
Marin County Division of Aging-AAA – San Rafael, CA
Monterey County Area Agency on Aging – Salinas, CA
Office on Aging-County of Orange – Santa Ana, CA
PASSAGES Adult Resource Center AAA – Chico, CA
Riverside County Office on Aging – Riverside, CA
San Diego County AAA – San Diego, CA
San Francisco Department of Aging and Adult Services –
    San Francisco, CA
San Mateo County AAA – San Mateo, CA
Sonoma County AAA Adult and Aging Services Division –
    Santa Rosa, CA
Stanislaus County AAA CA – Modesto, CA
Ventura County AAA – Ventura, CA

Colorado

Boulder County Aging Services Division – Boulder, CO
Denver Regional Council of Governments – Denver, CO
East Central Colorado AAA – Stratton, CO
Larimer County Office on Aging – Fort Collins, CO
NW Colorado Council of Governments – Silverthorne, CO
Region 10 AAA – Montrose, CO
South Central Council of Governments – Trinidad, CO
Upper Arkansas AAA – Salida, CO

Connecticut

Agency on Aging of South Central Connecticut, Inc –
    New Haven, CT
Eastern Connecticut AAA – Norwich, CT
North Central AAA Inc. – Hartford, CT
Southwestern Connecticut Agency on Aging – Bridgeport, CT
Western Connecticut Area Agency on Aging, Inc –
    Waterbury, CT

Florida

AAA for North Florida Inc. – Tallahassee, FL
AAA of Palm Beach/Treasure Coast Inc. – West Palm Beach, FL
Area Agency on Aging for SW Florida, Inc. – Fort Myers, FL
Elder Options – Gainesville, FL
Northeast Florida AAA Inc. – Jacksonville, FL
Northwest Florida AAA – Pensacola, FL
West Central Florida AAA Inc. – Tampa, FL

Georgia

Atlanta Regional Commission Aging Services Division –
    Atlanta, GA
Central Savannah River Area Regional Development C –
    Augusta, GA
Coastal Georgia Regional Development Center – Brunswick, GA
Coosa Valley RDC – Rome, GA
Lower Chattahoochee AAA – Columbus, GA
Middle Georgia RDC/AAA – Macon, GA
Northeast Georgia AAA – Athens, GA
Southeast Georgia RDC – Waycross, GA
Southern Crescent AAA – Franklin, GA
The Legacy Link Inc. – Gainesville, GA

Hawaii

Elderly Affairs Division – Honolulu, HI
Maui County Office on Aging – Wailuku, HI

Idaho

Area VI Agency on Aging – Idaho Falls, ID
College of Southern Idaho – Twin Falls, ID
North Central Idaho AAA – Lewiston, ID
North Idaho College/Area Agency on Aging – Coeur d' Alene, ID
Southwest Idaho AAA @ Sage Community Resources –
    Garden City, ID

Illinois

AgeOptions – Oak Park, IL
Area Agency on Aging for Lincolnland – Springfield, IL
Area Agency on Aging of Southwestern Illinois – Belleville, IL
East Central Illinois AAA – Bloomington, IL
Egyptian AAA – Carterville, IL
Northeastern Illinois AAA – Kankakee, IL
Northwestern Illinois AAA – Rockford, IL
Western Illinois AAA – Rock Island, IL

Indiana

Aging & In-Home Services of Northeast Indiana Inc. –
    Fort Wayne, IN
Area 10 Agency on Aging – Ellettsville, IN
Area 9 In-Home and Community Service Agency – Richmond, IN
Area IV Agency on Aging & Community Services – Lafayette, IN
CICOA Aging & In-Home Solutions, Inc. – Indianapolis, IN
Generations Area 13 Agency on Aging – Vincennes, IN
LifeSpan Resources, Inc – New Albany, IN
LifeStream Services, Inc. – Yorktown, IN
LifeTime Resources – Dillsboro, IN

Iowa

Aging Resources of Central Iowa – Des Moines, IA
Generations Area Agency on Aging – Davenport, IA
Hawkeye Valley AAA – Waterloo, IA
Northland Agency on Aging – Decorah, IA
Northwest Aging Association – Spencer, IA
Scenic Valley Area VIII AAA – Dubuque, IA
Seneca Area Agency on Aging – Ottumwa, IA
Siouxland Aging Services Inc. – Sioux City, IA
Southwest 8 Senior Services Inc. – Council Bluffs, IA
The Heritage Agency – Cedar Rapids, IA

Kansas

Central Plains AAA – Wichita, KS
East Central Kansas AAA – Ottawa, KS
North Central-Flint Hill AAA – Manhattan, KS
Southwest Kansas AAA – Dodge City, KS

Kentucky

Barren River Area Agency on Aging – Bowling Green, KY
Big Sandy Area Development District – Prestonsburg, KY
Bluegrass AAA – Lexington, KY
Buffalo Trace AAA – Maysville, KY
Gateway Area Development District – Morehead, KY
Green River AAA – Owensboro, KY
Kentuckiana Regional Planning and Development Agency –
   Louisville, KY
Lake Cumberland AAA – Russell Springs, KY
Lincoln Trail AAA – Elizabethtown, KY
North Kentucky Area Development District – Florence, KY

Louisiana

Caddo Council on Aging Inc. – Shreveport, LA
Caldwell Parish Council on Aging – Columbia, LA
Capital AAA – Baton Rouge, LA
Coast Council on Aging St. Tammy – Covington, LA
Jefferson Council on Aging Inc. – Metairie, LA
Lafourche Council on Aging – Raceland, LA
Terrebonne Council on Aging Inc. – Houma, LA

Maine

Central Maine AAA/Spectrum Generations – Augusta, ME
Eastern Agency on Aging – Bangor, ME
SeniorsPlus – Lewiston, ME
Southern Maine AAA Inc. – Scarborough, ME

Maryland

Baltimore City Commission on Aging Retirement Education –
Baltimore, MD
Frederick County Department on Aging – Frederick, MD
Montgomery County AAA – Rockville, MD
St. Mary's County Department of Aging – Leonardtown, MD

Massachusetts

BayPath Elder Services, Inc – Marlborough, MA
Boston Commission on Affairs of the Elderly – Boston, MA
Central Massachusetts Agency on Aging – W. Boylston, MA
Coastline Elderly Services Inc. – New Bedford, MA
Elder Services of Berkshire County Inc. – Pittsfield, MA
Elder Services of Cape Cod & the Islands – South Dennis, MA
Elder Services of Merrimack Valley Inc. – Lawrence, MA
Greater Lynn Senior Services – Lynn, MA
Greater Springfield Senior Services Inc. – Springfield, MA
Health & Social Services Consortium Inc. – Sharon, MA
Highland Valley Elder Services – Florence, MA
Mystic Valley Elder Services – Malden, MA
North Shore Elder Services Inc. – Danvers, MA
SeniorCare Inc. – Gloucester, MA
Somerville-Cambridge Elder Services – Somerville, MA
Springwell, Inc – Watertown, MA
WestMass ElderCare Inc. – Holyoke, MA

Michigan

AAA 1-B – Southfield, MI
AAA of Northwest Michigan – Traverse City, MI
Detroit AAA – Detroit, MI
Northeast Michigan Community Services Agency – Alpena, MI
Region 2 AAA – Brooklyn, MI
Region IV AAA – Saint Joseph, MI
Region VII AAA – Bay City, MI
Senior Resources of West Michigan/AAA – Muskegon Heights, MI

The Senior Alliance/AAA 1-C – Wayne, MI
Tri-County Office on Aging – Lansing, MI
Upper Peninsula AAA – Escanaba, MI
Valley AAA – Flint, MI

Minnesota

Arrowhead AAA – Duluth, MN
Central Minnesota Council on Aging – St. Cloud, MN
Metropolitan AAA – North St. Paul, MN
Minnesota River AAA – Mankato, MN

Mississippi

SMPDD Area Agency on Aging – Gulfport, MS

Missouri

Care Connection for Aging Services – Warrensburg, MO
Central Missouri AAA – Columbia, MO
Mid-East Area Agency on Aging – Manchester, MO
Southeast Missouri AAA – Cape Girardeau, MO
Southwest Missouri Office on Aging – Springfield, MO

New Jersey

Bergen County Division of Senior Services – Hackensack, NJ
Hunterdon County Office on Aging – Flemington, NJ
Somerset County Office on Aging – Somerville, NJ
Union County Division on Aging – Elizabeth, NJ

New Mexico

City of Albuquerque AAA – Albuquerque, NM

New York

Allegany County Office for the Aging – Belmont, NY
At Regis Mohawk Tribe Office for the Aging – Hogansburg, NY
Batavia-Genesee Senior Center – Batavia, NY
Broome County Office for Aging – Binghamton, NY

Cattaraugus County Dept. of Aging – Olean, NY
Chemung County Department of Aging and Long Term C –
Elmira, NY
Clinton County Office for the Aging – Plattsburgh, NY
Cortland County AAA – Cortland, NY
Delaware County Office for the Aging – Delhi, NY
Dutchess County Office for the Aging – Poughkeepsie, NY
Erie County Dept. of Senior Services – Buffalo, NY
Fulton County Office for Aging – Johnstown, NY
Livingston County Office for Aging – Mt. Morris, NY
Madison County Office for the Aging – Canastota, NY
Monroe County Office for the Aging – Rochester, NY
Montgomery County Office for the Aging – Amsterdam, NY
New York City Department for the Aging – New York, NY
Onondaga County Dept. of Aging & Youth – Syracuse, NY
Orleans County Office for the Aging – Albion, NY
Rensselaer County Dept. for the Aging – Troy, NY
Rockland County Office for the Aging – Pomona, NY
St. Lawrence County Office for the Aging – Canton, NY
Steuben County Office for the Aging – Bath, NY
TIOGA Opportunities, Department of Aging – Owego, NY
Ulster County Office for the Aging – Kingston, NY
Westchester County Department of Senior Programs & –
Mount Vernon, NY
Wyoming County Office for Aging – Warsaw, NY

North Carolina
Area Agency on Aging – Wilmington, NC
High Country AAA – Boone, NC
Land of Sky Regional Council – Asheville, NC
Northwest Piedmont Council of Governments – Winston-Salem, NC
Piedmont Triad Council of Governments AAA – Greensboro, NC
Southwestern Commission AAA – Sylva, NC
Triangle J Council of Governments – Research Triangle Park, NC
Upper Coastal Plain Council of Governments – Rocky Mount, NC

Western Piedmont Council of Governments/AAA – Hickory, NC

Ohio

AAA 10B, Inc. – Uniontown, OH
AAA District 7 Inc. – Rio Grande, OH
AAA PSA #2 – Dayton, OH
AAA PSA #3 – Lima, OH
AAA Region 9 Inc. – Byesville, OH
Area Office on Aging of Northwestern Ohio Inc. – Toledo, OH
Buckeye Hills AAA – Reno, OH
Central Ohio AAA-City of Columbus – Columbus, OH
Council on Aging of Southwestern Ohio – Cincinnati, OH
District XI Area Agency on Aging, Inc. – Youngstown, OH
Ohio District 5 AAA – Mansfield, OH
Western Reserve AAA – Cleveland, OH

Oklahoma

AAA Eastern Oklahoma Development District – Muskogee, OK
Absentee-Shawnee Tribe – Shawnee, OK
COEDD AAA – Shawnee, OK
Grand Gateway AAA – Big Cabin, OK
NODA – Enid, OK
South Western Oklahoma Development Authority – Burns Flat, OK
Tulsa AAA – Tulsa, OK

Oregon

Central Oregon Council on Aging – Redmond, OR
Douglas County Senior Services Division – Roseburg, OR
Multnomah County Aging and Disability Services Div –
    Portland, OR
NorthWest Senior & Disability Services – Salem, OR
Oregon Cascades West Council of Governments – Albany, OR
Rogue Valley Council of Governments Senior & Disability
    Program – Central Point, OR
Senior and Disabled Services, Lane COG – Eugene, OR

Washington County Disability, Aging & Veteran Services –
Hillsboro, OR

Pennsylvania

Cambria County AAA – Johnstown, PA
Chester County Dept. of Aging Services – West Chester, PA
Greater Erie Community Action Committee – Erie, PA
Lancaster County Office of Aging – Lancaster, PA
Lehigh County AAA – Allentown, PA
Montgomery County Aging & Adult Services – Norristown, PA
Philadelphia Corporation for Aging – Philadelphia, PA
Schuylkill County Office of Senior Services – Pottsville, PA
Venango County AAA – Franklin, PA
York County AAA – York, PA

South Carolina

Catawba AAA – Rock Hill, SC
Central Midlands Council of Governments – Columbia, SC
Lower Savannah Council of Governments – Aiken, SC
South Carolina Appalachian Council of Governments –
Greenville, SC
Vantage Point-Division of CareSouth Carolina, Inc. – Hartsville, SC

Tennessee

First Tennessee AAA – Johnson City, TN
Greater Nashville AAA – Nashville, TN
South Central Tennessee Development District/AAA –
Columbia, TN
Southwest AAAD – Jackson, TN

Texas

AAA of Southeast Texas – Beaumont, TX
AAA of the Panhandle – Amarillo, TX
Alamo Area Council of Governments/AAA – San Antonio, TX
Area Agency on Aging of the Capital Area – Austin, TX

Ark-Tex Council of Governments/Area Agency on Aging – Texarkana, TX

Bexar County Area Agency on Aging – San Antonio, TX

Coastal Bend AAA – Corpus Christi, TX

Concho Valley Council of Governments/AAA – San Angelo, TX

Dallas AAA – Dallas, TX

Deep East Texas Council of Governments/AAA – Jasper, TX

East Texas AAA – Kilgore, TX

Heart of Texas AAA – Waco, TX

Houston-Galveston Area Council – Houston, TX

Houston-Harris County AAA – Houston, TX

Lower Rio Grande Valley AAA – McAllen, TX

Middle Rio Grande AAA – Carrizo Springs, TX

Permian Basin AAA – Midland, TX

Rio Grande Council of Governments – El Paso, TX

South Plains Association of Governments – Lubbock, TX

Utah

5 County AAA – St. George, UT

Davis County Senior Services – Farmington, UT

Salt Lake County Aging Services – Salt Lake, UT

Vermont

AAA for Northeastern Vermont – St. Johnsbury, VT

Central Vermont Council on Aging – Barre, VT

Champlain Valley Agency on Aging, Inc – Winooski, VT

Council on Aging for Southeastern Vermont Inc. – Springfield, VT

Southwestern Vermont Council on Aging – Rutland, VT

Virginia

Alexandria Agency on Aging – Alexandria, VA

Arlington AAA – Arlington, VA

Bay Aging – Urbanna, VA

Central Virginia AAA – Lynchburg, VA

Crater District AAA – Petersburg, VA

Fairfax AAA – Fairfax, VA
LOA AAA Inc. – Roanoke, VA
Mountain Empire Older Citizens Inc. – Big Stone Gap, VA
Prince William AAA – Manassas, VA
Rappahannock AAA – Fredericksburg, VA
Rappahannock-Rapidan Community Services Board –
    Culpeper, VA
Senior Connections – Richmond, VA
Senior Services of Southeastern Virginia – Norfolk, VA
Shenandoah AAA – Front Royal, VA
Southern AAA Inc. – Martinsville, VA

Washington

Aging & Adult Care of Central Washington – E. Wenatchee, WA
Lewis/Mason/Thurston AAA – Olympia, WA
Northwest Washington AAA – Bellingham, WA
Olympic AAA – Port Hadlock, WA
Pierce County Human Services – Tacoma, WA
Seattle/King County Area Agency on Aging – Seattle, WA
Southeast Washington Aging and LTC – Yakima, WA

West Virginia

Northwestern AAA–Bel-O-Mar Regional Council/Planning –
    Wheeling, WV

Wisconsin

AAA of Dane County – Madison, WI
AgeAdvantAge, Inc – Madison, WI
Bay AAA – Green Bay, WI
Milwaukee County Department on Aging – Milwaukee, WI
Northern Area Agency on Aging Inc. – Rhinelander, WI
Southeastern AAA – Brookfield, WI

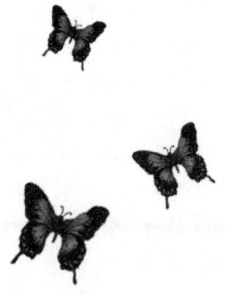

About the Author

Frena Gray-Davidson was born and raised in England. She worked as a feature writer and broadcaster in Asia for fifteen years and was the NBC Radio Correspondent for Nepal. In Hong Kong, she studied Chinese medicine and acupuncture for five years, as well as Tai Chi. She came to the USA in 1986, where she first become involved in Alzheimer's care.

She has been a support group facilitator for the Alzheimer's Association, keynote speaker for the Royal Alzheimer Society of Great Britain, and has trained professional dementia-care workers and educated family caregivers for over ten years. She is the author of seventeen books, including *The Book of Chinese Beliefs* and *Ayurvedic Healing*. She also wrote *The Alzheimer's Sourcebook*, now in its third edition, described by Dr. Tom Kitwood of the groundbreaking Bradford Dementia Project as "the best book on Alzheimer's I've ever read."

Frena is an international presenter of workshops on dementia. She currently resides in Bisbee, Arizona. You can email her at frenagd@juno.com. Check out her webpage at www.alzguide.com.

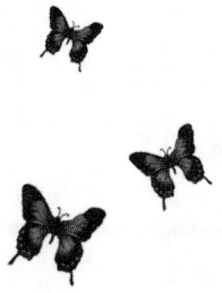

Other Books By
Frena Gray-Davidson

<u>as Frena Gray-Davidson</u>

Rough Tao
The Alzheimer's Sourcebook
Alzheimer's FAQ
The Caregiver's Sourcebook
Ayurvedic Healing

<u>as Frena Bloomfield</u>

Book of Chinese Beliefs
Harmony Rules: A Guide to Chinese Medicine
Healing Plants: Ginseng
Healing Plants: Aloe Vera
Odyssey Guide to Sri Lanka
Odyssey Guide to Thailand
The Skyfleet of Atlantis
The Guardian of the Dragon Paths

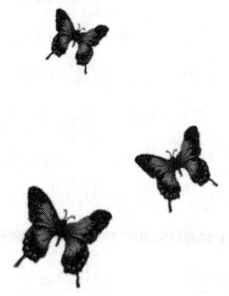

Endorsements for Frena's Other Books

"This book is a *must have* for caregivers or anyone who has a family member with Alzheimer's. You can read it through or just pick out chapters that will help you at the time, but the biggest help to me was Chapter 12 about Approaching Death. It gave me the comfort and help that I needed. I've read many books on the subject, but this has been the most helpful yet because it is based on love."

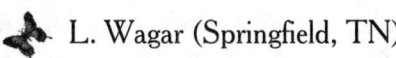 — L. Wagar (Springfield, TN)

Great Learning Tool

"For anyone with a loved one suffering with Alzheimer's this is the book to get. It will help you understand the disease and how to cope. Written in everyday language it is packed with information on the stages these victims go through and how you can help them. One of the best I've read!"

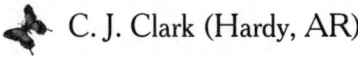 — C. J. Clark (Hardy, AR)

This Book Has the Answers You Are Looking For

"This is the book that changed everything for me. It's about approaching this disease with Love, Strength, and Courage. Frena shows you how to get thru a day at a time and most of all how to keep yourself intact. We get lost in this disease; it consumes whole families. She shows you how to listen; your loved one is still within this person afflicted by this disease. You just have to listen carefully and you will see the person you love is still inside and has a lot to tell. She shows you how to cope. Frena is my strength; she gave me the tools from reading her book three years ago. This book is my foundation and Frena is an angel. No other book affected me as much as this one. If you want to truly understand this disease, this is it!"

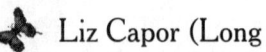 Liz Capor (Long Island, New York)

A Book that Packs a Powerful Message about Love

"This is a tremendous resource for people who believe in the healing power of Love. Frena Gray-Davidson has written a very spiritually centered book that will inevitably help any caregiver and their loved one."

She speaks about how we'll see the 'divine child' untouched by darkness or sickness—our loved one—emerge in this process. And she states that we must listen to the feeling behind the words. That little statement has changed my life. When someone asks for their mother, who may have passed on decades earlier, they're really seeking comfort and security and reassurance. We need to hear their feelings that lie in back of their words."

She goes on to say that 30% of language is verbal; the rest is expressed in body language and behavior."

Further on she makes the observation that Alzheimer's patients are sensitive to the thoughts of those around them and to always give plenty of Love, both in word, action and thought."

She states that 'unconditional Love is not a measure; it is a flow. You cannot give it or get it; you can only be part of it. When you love a person with Alzheimers, clarity and awareness come to that person.'"

"The other wonderful point she makes is that so much of our disappointment in Alzheimer's patients is tied to our notion of their 'proper' mortal identity.

Your mother doesn't know she's your mother anymore, but you can value and cherish who she is in the here and now. Don't live in the past but nurture the childlike qualities she is expressing in the present."

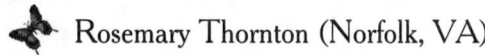 Rosemary Thornton (Norfolk, VA)

Your First-choice Book on Alzheimer's Disease

"Frena Gray-Davidson is the ultimate 'been there, done that' person in Alzheimer's care. Her book, *The Alzheimer's Sourcebook for Caregivers,* is a support group that can always be with you, ready to speak to the issues that concern you now and prepare you for what is likely to concern you in the future. All parts of this book will help you meet the challenges of dementia care; however several chapters are of special value. Chapter 2, Before Diagnosis and Chapter 4, Family Crisis Alzheimer's Style, guide families in the early stages of the disease. Chapter 11, Knowing When To Let Go, answers some of the tough questions about placement in a care facility. The final chapter, Moving On, gives guidance for that time when caregiving is no longer the top priority. In keeping with her theme not to lose the person in the process of coping with the disease, Ms. Gray-Davidson leads us away from using psychiatric terms to label behaviors and thought patterns which result from diminishing cognitive ability. She explains what may look like paranoia as 'a reasonable fear response, given the limitations of the disease.' She makes what is often labeled delusional thinking easier to understand as 'memory which has drifted into some point in the past.' She writes with compassion and humor, creating therapy for the caregiver and family members. The book is interesting to read and easy to understand. As a Geriatric Care Consultant, I have often loaned my copy of *The Alzheimer's Sourcebook for Caregivers* to my clients. Most of them return it with the comment that they have purchased copies for themselves and for family members. This started with the 1st edition and is continuing with the 3rd. I can make no higher recommendation."

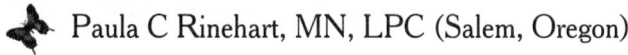 Paula C Rinehart, MN, LPC (Salem, Oregon)

Robert D. Reed Publishers Order Form

Call in your order for fast service and quantity discounts!
(541) 347- 9882

OR order on-line at **www.rdrpublishers.com** *using PayPal.*
OR order by FAX at **(541) 347-9883** *OR by mail:*
Make a copy of this form; enclose payment information:
Robert D. Reed Publishers
1380 Face Rock Drive, Bandon, OR 97411

Send indicated books to:

Name_____

Address_____

City_____ State _____ Zip _____

Phone: _____ Fax _____ Cell _____

E-Mail _____

Payment by check /_/ or credit card /_/ (All major credit cards are accepted.)

Name on card _____

Card Number _____

Exp. Date _____ Last 3-Digit number on back of card _____

	Quantity	Total Amount
Alzheimer's 911 by Frena Gray-Davidson $16.95	_____	_____
Travels in Place: A Journey into Memory Loss by Christiane W. Griffin-Wehr............................ $16.95	_____	_____
Liberty's Quest: The Compelling Story of the Wife and Mother of Two Poetry Pulitzer Prize Winners, James Wright and Franz Wright by Liberty Kovacs.......................... $29.95	_____	_____
Daily Intentions by Ann Blakely Rice................. $19.95	_____	_____
A.D.D. The 20-Hour Solution by Mark Steinberg, Ph.D.................................... $14.95	_____	_____
A Kid's Herb Book: For Children of All Ages by Lesley Tierra... $19.95	_____	_____

Quantity of books ordered: _____ Total amount for books: _____

Shipping is $3.50 1st book + $1 for each additional book: Plus postage: _____

FINAL TOTAL: _____